THE LAST CHANCE DOG

AND OTHER STORIES OF HOLISTIC ANIMAL HEALING

Donna Kelleher, D.V.M.

SCRIBNER

New York London Toronto Sydney Singapore

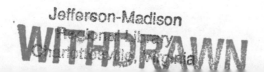

SCRIBNER
1230 Avenue of the Americas
New York, NY 10020

For information about special discounts for bulk purchases,
please contact Simon & Schuster Special Sales:
1-800-456-6798 or business@simonandschuster.com

DESIGNED BY ERICH HOBBING

Text set in Bembo

Manufactured in the United States of America

1   3   5   7   9   10   8   6   4   2

Library of Congress Cataloging-in-Publication Data
Kelleher, Donna.
The last chance dog : and other stories of holistic animal healing / Donna Kelleher.
p. cm.
Includes bibliographical references (p.)
1. Kelleher, Donna. 2. Veterinarians—Washington (State)—Seattle—Biography.
3. Women veterinarians—Washington (State)—Seattle—Biography.
4. Dogs—Washington (State)—Seattle—Anecdotes.
5. Cats—Washington (State)—Seattle—Anecdotes.
6. Pets—Washington (State)—Seattle—Anecdotes.
7. Holistic veterinary medicine—Washington (State)—Seattle—Anecdotes.
I. Title.
SF613.K43 A3 2003
636.089'55—dc21   2002030998

ISBN 0-7432-2301-2

To my grandmothers,
Ruth and Evelyn,
for whom giving love is second nature.
And to the animals who continuously teach me,
especially my own:
Smudge, Sugar, Charlie, and Igor.

CONTENTS

INTRODUCTION

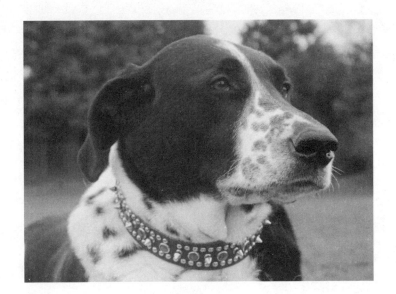

Seizures racked Sierra's long slinky body and she jiggled uncontrollably, flopping across the exam room floor. The staff at Seattle's Bird and Exotic Clinic frantically tried to catch her to prevent injury, but she wriggled free. Blood tests and radiographs indicated to Dr. Tracy Bennett that the patient might have suffered trauma, though no bones were broken. The seizures might have been less violent if Sierra had limbs; she might have been able to brace herself against the raging fits that slammed her body. But unfortunately, arms and legs are not part of her anatomy. Sierra is a ball python.

I transferred my knowledge of the canine Chinese meridians to Sierra and used acupuncture to treat what I believed, from a traditional Chinese medical point of view, to be Blood Stagnation. An hour later, the small snake lay still, resting her head in my palm with three acupuncture needles in place while the rest of her soft slippery body coiled loosely on the table. Her only movement was the repetitive inquisitive flicking of her tongue— a good sign, I was told. The seizures ceased, which thrilled the technicians as they had better things to do than chase down a seizing snake.

Lilly came in a few months later. Instead of ambling along like other lizards, she moved with her left front leg frozen straight behind her. As bearded dragons go, Lilly was a friendly sort, but her pain put her in the foulest of moods. The radiologist's report confirmed which joints were arthritic. Using information from the radiographs, along with my Chinese diagnosis of Bony Bi Syndrome, I treated her with acupuncture. Lilly rolled a prehistoric eye my way as I threaded tiny Korean hand needles into four points on her leg and foot. She was obviously sizing up my abilities as I surprised her even more by stimulating points with a laser. A few days later, she could bend her leg more easily. The swelling was down, and her mood had improved too, or at least that is what Mark Lee, her owner, said in his Cockney accent: "She's been a 'air more lively, I'd 'ave t' say."

Dyna is a bay pony who had always been a good communicator and, indeed, when she bucked her teenage rider off, she was attempting to tell the world that her back hurt. A typically even-tempered soul, now Dyna repetitively pinned her ears and kicked her back feet as high as she could off the ground. I did a chiropractic exam, and nearly every joint of her spine was fixed instead of flexible. After adjusting her and massaging her spasmed back muscles the next day, I saw that Dyna was as good as new, ready to jump again.

I never dreamed I would be using acupuncture or chiropractic for any animal, much less a snake or a lizard. But compassion tends to open the mind—I vowed to treat my patients as I would want to be treated, with respect for the body's innate ability to heal itself. For the seizing snake, stiff lizard, and bucking pony, the situation was the same—holistic medicine was simply the best treatment. Western medicine is great for diagnostic tests and treating certain surgical or critical patients, but for the vast majority of chronic diseases, there is a world of treatment options beyond antibiotics and anti-inflammatories.

Holistic medicine is the gentle medicine I longed to learn about in conventional veterinary school. I found myself asking whether the scientific approach could be more compassionate toward the body and spirit. All prescription drugs have side effects. Drug companies go to great lengths to prove their products are safe, but the fact remains that those studies, whether they are on new vaccines or other drugs, are short in duration compared to the life of an animal or a person. Conversely, over thousands of years most forms of natural medicine have been proved to be safe.

This is good medicine for the whole planet. Since we rely on naturally derived plant materials and support only small independent companies, natural-medicine practitioners tread more lightly on our environment. Many of us generate less disposable, plastic medical waste. Holistic medicine is safer on our bodies as well. It helps the body to repair itself with far fewer side effects than occur with pharmaceutical drugs. When we treat both ourselves and our pets with natural medicine, we can live a healthier and longer life.

Come join me on my journey into holistic veterinary medicine. The chapters of my book follow my career from animal-emergency practice into the world of holistic medicine. I listen to the animals, peer into their souls, tell their stories, and heal them. Each chapter highlights a new animal and a new natural method of treatment and raises philosophical questions about the veterinary profession.

You, the concerned pet owners, have the power to change the way we think about and treat animals. If you ask for natural medicines, more veterinarians will offer them. If you demand that veterinary colleges incorporate well-proven treatments such as acupuncture and chiropractic, the veterinary curriculum will change, however slowly. Learning the first step toward a more compassionate way to treat your beloved winged, scaled, or furry pet is here—right in your hands.

GOODBYE ANIMAL ER

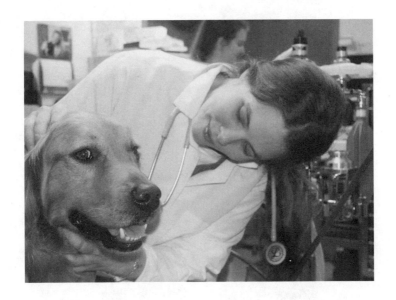

Emergency medicine always caused a rush of emotions. Once, I remember, a golden retriever came in with a foot-long laceration spanning the width of his chest. I spent three hours stitching him back together. His owners called me two weeks later to say he was as good as new. I loved every time a tiny, comatose kitten popped back to his feet after I gave him a few drops of sugar solution and warmed him up. Usually, after I treated those kittens for parasites, dehydration, and anorexia, they miraculously recuperated. But over time, I began to worry about each animal who was not improving. Eventually, this worry dragged down my healing energies like weights around my ankles.

Early one warm June evening, I'd found it difficult to come in to work for the whole night when the sun told me it was still afternoon. I had just walked into the clinic when Tanya, the technician, greeted me with one of those "Oh no, this is going to be bad" looks. There was an old black lab in exam room one, and as I entered the white sterile room, a strange, loud, odd symphony of chewing struck me. With a twist of the stomach, I realized that it sounded like a movie theater audience stuffing their faces with popcorn.

I looked at the patient. She was lying on her side in the bottom of a plastic travel crate and was unable to get up or even raise her head. She was thin, dehydrated, and sad, and I felt sure the spirit world had forgotten to send for her. I was so shocked to see her in such miserable condition that I forgot momentarily about investigating the origin of the chewing sound.

The dog's owner was an older, seemingly well-off woman with a thick gold bracelet, and a matching necklace below her freshly bobbed hair. "Why did you wait so long to bring her in?" I snapped. I knew it was good, at least, that she had come in, but it was hard to stay composed. My hands began to shake.

She shrugged and sighed. "My son was supposed to be caring for her while we were in Europe." Her words were awkward and abrupt, leaving me to wonder later whether she was more traumatized than her cool demeanor suggested.

I absentmindedly ran my hand along the dog's back while I listened to the woman's excuses. Suddenly, a large clump of what had been skin fell into my hand, revealing the source of those haunting chewing sounds. Thousands of maggots were making the poor paralyzed dog's back their home. These fly larvae set up shop on immobile animals that sit in their own excrement; they had burrowed deeply into both of the dog's hind legs and even into her abdominal cavity. They swirled and wriggled at the disturbance.

Startled, I stepped back for a second. "I'm sorry," I said, filled with sympathy for this forlorn creature but wanting to strangle the woman. "At this point, there is little we can do for her except euthanize her." I could hardly believe I was saying those words, but they came to me quickly, without hesitation.

Outwardly, she did not seem upset. She shed no tears, and her eyes were cool and focused. "I knew you'd say that," she replied sharply. She looked down at the floor. "Where do I pay?" she said abruptly. The woman left, without turning to say goodbye to her dog. Perhaps she was too embarrassed, or hardened. I wondered if I saw tears confined to the corners of her eyes in the final instant when we made unavoidable eye contact. She might have been wondering how *her own son* could treat another living being this way.

Tanya and I returned to the plastic crate and the dog nestled within it. She looked through me with a miserable gaze, unable to move. I knew she could read my intent as I kneeled to give her a sedative injection. I felt she knew I was going to end her suffering. Animals may not dwell on death as people do, but they do know pain. I felt the transfer of her pain into me in the form of nausea as I injected the thick pink euthanasia solution into a vein on her front leg. As I euthanized her, I thought I felt her spirit lick my cheek as she bounded into her next life. A little while later, since they had also ingested the deadly solution, the maggots finally ceased their terrible chatter.

The cold steel and white walls that surrounded me now were a far cry from the farms, the fields, and the horses who had originally drawn me toward animals and eventually into veterinary medicine. Sometimes as veterinarians go through life we realize that what drew us to help is lost, that our dream of curing animals has become clouded over—not by dark influences, but by a toughness that develops over time. I had gone through vet school and had been a practicing dog and cat emergency vet for five years when it finally dawned on me: I was not on the right path.

Late that night, on duty at the ER, I slept on a hard dusty futon crammed into the bathroom to shut out the sting of the bright fluorescent lights. I dreamed about living in England more than ten years earlier, when I'd first thought of becoming a veterinarian; I remembered those months spent in horse boot camp fondly, even though the sagging mattresses had been no more comfortable than this one.

Many memories have stuck with me from the nearly two years I spent in England training to be a horseback riding instructor. White sheep speckled the green rolling hills surrounding the cobblestone and brick horse stable where I trained. Since I have been around horses all my life, I can't smell horse manure but I sure remember the piercing smell of sheep dung every morning. I recall the purple face of my stern and stout instructor, Carole, as she shouted orders. Most of all, I remember Fiona Wainwright's bright red hair bobbing against the deep green of the beautiful fields of western Dorset. Our trails had been trodden upon for hundreds of years and Fiona and I would ride along hedgerows and stone fences whenever we could sneak away from our busy barnyard schedule. Fiona was a fellow British Horse Society student instructor who did not share my fear of jumping.

My memory of my first day at the Dorset School of Equitation is one I'll always treasure, the way one fondly remembers things that, at the time, were definitely no fun—like losing baby teeth. I remember Carole pulling my body into a new position she thought would improve my jumping. I was standing in the middle of the arena on a nice ex-event horse named Sam, who seemed thoroughly bored with the whole heated conversation. "No, not like that!" Carole grabbed my riding pants to scoot my bottom back the way the British jump. "Bring your hips back over the saddle. You bloody Americans jump too far forward." I noticed, as the other girls would later concur, how Carole's purple lips bulged and her posture grew more rigid the more aggravated she became. I wasn't sure if it was my new riding position or my nervousness, but as I approached the three-and-a-half-foot jump, in slow motion, the earth became the sky and I tumbled off the horse, hitting the ground with a loud thud.

In that moment, as I sat stunned in the dirt, I heard a voice, maybe an old riding instructor or maybe my mother from years ago, tell me, "Donna, falling is something you are good at. People learn a lot from falling." It was true. As I fell, instead of clenching to fight the fall, my body had instinctively relaxed, as if I were bareback on my cousin's farm again arguing a no-win battle with the old barnyard pony Flicka, who fortunately was short enough that the falls were less painful. It was a simple argument: she wanted to go to the barn and I wanted to go riding into the field. She would buck and swerve and buck and eventually lie down until she had pinned my seven-year-old body to the ground. Round over: Pony wins again. But my mother would coach me, into the twilight, from on top of a tattered toolshed overlooking the barnyard. Comforted by the summer night sparkle of blinking fireflies, through tears and turmoil she would make sure, at least, that I got back on, no matter what.

My mother's coaching taught me to search for my own truth. While growing up, I listened to her discuss her work as an international studies professor. We had visitors from other countries who ate, spoke, and treated their medical ailments differently than we did. I learned that the conventional American way was not necessarily the best way—that we all see the world through only our own narrow window of experience. Many years later, when I found myself in my first year of veterinary school with formaldehyde-induced nosebleeds from spending so much time with preserved dog cadavers for anatomy class, I called my mother for advice.

One time my mother and I went hiking, near vet school in eastern Washington, with my little black dog. I had rescued Smudge, but her emotional turmoil had scarred her to the point of submissive urination. Veterinarians always seem to own abnormal animals with complicated histories. "How can my classmates kill normal pound dogs, bought for fifty dollars, supposedly just to learn surgery?" I asked my mother. We were at the top of Kamiak Butte, overlooking the treeless rolling hills of the Palouse. She had no answer, and I guess I couldn't have expected one. I would have felt better about taking those lives if I'd believed that what students learned made up for it in some way. But I didn't feel sure of that. I decided to take alternative surgery, in which we performed procedures on dead animals euthanized for terminal illnesses. Headed by Dr. Karl White, the veterinary chool at Washington State University was known for its progressive non-kill surgery classes, and for that I was thankful. Otherwise I would not have made it through veterinary school.

During one of my most difficult nights at vet school, I was on rotation with Teresa, now a racetrack vet, who was always tougher than I was, more the way I thought an equine vet should be. We were walking a young former racehorse to prevent him from getting colic, a life-threatening stomachache horses experience because they can't vomit. Walking colicky horses helps keep their digestive tracts moving, and can even save their lives! The horse had probably come from a second-rate racetrack. It was obvious that he had had an awful life. As part of a research project on how drugs affect intestinal motility, one of our vet school teachers had done an experimental surgery on the horse. The sickly horse had hardly been an ideal surgery candidate; thin and crawling with lice, he had been acquired by the vet school via a horse trader.

Now, every time we students stopped walking him, he would attempt to lie down and roll on or kick at his stomach. We switched off who walked him, as we had been told to do, and between us, we kept him moving and medicated all night. I turned to see his face in the moonlight. His body was coated with sweat, and his terror-filled eyes showed their white outlines bright against his dark body. His legs were riddled with scars, knobs, and bumps, evidence of life on the track. Even though he would rather have lain down, he followed each of us obediently, as thoroughbreds have been bred to do.

When Teresa walked the horse, she did not complain; with each step, she seemed more complacent, more resigned to the fact that it didn't matter what she thought, anyway. I screamed at her from over the fence, "This sucks! He should have known not to cut this one," and numerous other colorful complaints lent to me by my fiery Irish heritage, a habit that hadn't won me any brownie points with the powers that govern a veterinary college.

But I knew that people like Teresa fit in well at the racetrack. All these years I'd looked up to her because she was a hard scientist, so interesting and tough. Through vet school, her freezer was filled with roadkill to be studied and dissected. Her shelves were decorated with skeletons of snakes, possums, and raccoons. I loved her like a sister, but as I watched her calmly lead the pained horse by his tattered rope, I knew that my veterinary career would need to move in a more compassionate direction.

I wondered if there was a safer way to treat animals through the veterinary curriculum. Discussions about "iatrogenic" (doctor-induced) disease worried me. Why should *we* be the cause of any disease? These questions festered within my consciousness, but when I looked around, most of the other students didn't seem to share my concerns. They might have been more concerned with the next exam.

I knew from my years with horses that sticking with it through difficult times would be worthwhile. In vet school, I felt as if I were falling off a horse again. Eventually, I thought, if I dusted myself off enough times, like with Sam in England and Flicka in the old barnyard in New York, I would be pleased with my endurance. I believed that when I graduated and began working as a veterinarian in the real world, I would love my job. But that night on ER I felt like I was still falling.

At 1:00 A.M. we got the call most ER vets have come to dread. Tanya came to tell me, "A breeder is on the phone. She says her boxer is straining but can't have her puppies. She's on her way in." Nervous twinges began churning in my stomach as I checked to make sure all the surgical equipment needed for a C-section was sterilized and ready to go.

Tanya warned me after she left the exam room that this was going to be a difficult breeder. When I entered the room, I saw the boxer bitch on the floor, pushing, with no results. "She needs a C-section, just like last year," the breeder ordered.

"How old is she?" I asked, resenting being pushed into anything, since it's my veterinary license on the line.

"Seven, and been bred every year of her life. I've made thousands of dollars from her puppies. I would have gone to my regular vet, but he's out of town," she said in a snippy tone, as if she were trying to annoy me.

"Well, because of her history, I hate to rush right into surgery," I said. "I'd like to take a radiograph and try an oxytocin injection first."

"I guess, but it's a waste of time. How many C-sections have you done? You couldn't be more than twenty-five years old." She leaned forward, staring right at me. Although there are responsible breeders, they never seemed to come in on my shift. I questioned the idea of breeding dogs when less high-strung, more unusual, and healthier mixed-breed dogs are euthanized every day in animal shelters.

"I've done quite a few, and I look young for my age." I hoped she would lay off. "If you want to go to another emergency clinic, by all means, we can refer you somewhere." An extended silence accompanied the building tension between us. Only the quiet hum of the fluorescent light above us filled the exam room. She sighed, resolved to let me handle things, and went home.

Unlike her owner, Madeline was very forgiving and kind-tempered. She groaned and tried to push a puppy out every few minutes, turning nervously to see if she had been successful. I took her over to the X-ray table. Tanya and I laughed a little, despite our unspoken stress, while we took her radiograph. "Well, at least she's nicer than that bulldog we had last week," Tanya said. Unlike boxers, by and large bulldogs can't give birth without C-sections.

"Yeah, but this breeder is a real gem," I said as we turned Madeline on her back for another view. My cynical East Coast side always became more pronounced in the middle of the night.

The radiographs showed that Madeline had six large puppies, and the one in the birth canal was positioned sideways. After putting some exam gloves on, I tried to turn the puppy around, while Madeline strained against my fingers. It was no use. I couldn't even feel the puppy; my fingers were too short. Oxytocin wouldn't help here, since the puppy was just too big for the canal.

Within ten minutes, due to Tanya's fast preparation, Madeline lay anesthetized, belly and snout up, all four feet tied to the corners of the steel table. With tubes and intravenous lines draped everywhere, I was already cutting her open with a scalpel blade. I felt as if Madeline knew the ropes better than I, having gone through all of this before so many times.

I had always said that surgery made me nervous, but at least C-sections were rewarding. I just hoped the puppies were alive. Madeline seemed so much older than seven. I used scissors to cut the wall of the uterus, which was scarred and very unhealthy because of the number of litters Madeline had endured. I squeezed the first puppy through a small hole in the uterus, and passed it to Tanya to resuscitate, amniotic sac and all. She caught the puppy in a towel and wiped it to stimulate and revive it, just as Madeline would have done if she had given birth by herself. "Looks like a little brindle girl," she said. We read one another's minds. This puppy's tan and brown color would ensure her survival. If she had been white, it would have been customary for her to be killed, either by the veterinarian who delivered her or by the breeder because of breed-standard biases.

One at a time, assembly-line style, I delivered and Tanya revived all six puppies: three girls and three boys. We had only one problem as we woke Madeline up from anesthesia. One little boy puppy was white. I didn't know what to do. Tanya suggested I keep it quiet. "Just don't tell her. You know what she'll say. We'll find him a home ourselves," she said.

If I were to take the puppy home and not inform the breeder, I could lose my license. Of course, euthanizing the puppy would be what she would want, and I wouldn't do that. *Maybe she'll be reasonable,* I thought. So against Tanya's wishes and my better judgment, over the phone I begged the breeder to take the puppy home.

"If you don't kill him, I will," the breeder snapped at me.

"I can't and won't do that," I said, but I was getting that nervous feeling in my stomach again. "I could find a home for him," I persisted. Many breeders don't even like that, because if the gossip spreads, the boxer community might think a breeder's bloodline is substandard. It's a dark secret. Some veterinarians turn a blind eye, facilitating life only to end it, becoming like the cold steel we hover over. Finally she said, "Okay. I can see you won't back down, so let's forget we ever had this conversation. I'll pick up the bitch and the other pups within the hour." I took that to mean we could save the white male, and I breathed a sigh of relief.

Tanya and I gloated over the white boy pup like he was ours, wrapping him in a towel and watching him wrinkle his face, sucking on a bottle. We thought it was sad that he wouldn't meet his mother, but we started to plan what we would do with him. I would make sure he got a great home.

The end of the night was approaching; as Madeline went home, I could see the blue light of early dawn on the horizon. Relieved to see this shift coming to an end, I went into the office to finish writing up my records. But at that moment Tanya came in, munching on a cookie, to tell me that we had a cat on its way.

A short while later, I met a very upset but thankfully kind elderly lady and her calico kitten in the exam room. The lady stood next to the exam table stroking her kitten, who was open-mouth breathing. "Please don't let her die," she begged. "I lost my husband last week to cancer and I really need Pounces now." She took the kitten into her arms and rocked her like a baby.

I quickly glanced at the kitten's medical record. "I see here that she had a vaccine yesterday. Was she sick before the vaccine?" Trained to remain objective, I had to brush aside for now the comments about her husband dying or my thinking would be even more clouded than it already was from another sleepless night. Pounces, herself, seemed confused about what was happening to her body; breathing took all her effort.

"No. She was her frisky self before yesterday, but after we came here, she vomited all night long," the woman said, fidgeting nervously with the yellow scarf tied tightly around her neck. I quickly examined the kitten. It was clear that the woman's distress was almost as great as her pet's. By her broken words, I knew that she felt the worst dread imaginable at the prospect of losing the small kitten who kept her house alive. I imagined Pounces climbing her curtains and springing from countertops to sofa backs, providing movement in a house that was now otherwise so still. Perhaps this little kitten was all that was keeping her going right now.

I knew saving the kitten would be a race against the clock. "I'll have to hurry up and treat her," I said. "Her temp. is 105 F, three degrees above normal, and I think she's having a vaccine reaction." *How dangerous vaccines can be,* I thought, but there was little time for thinking.

"I have to get started right away," I said anxiously to the woman, and noticed myself scratching my head even though it didn't itch—one of many nervous habits I didn't remember having before working emergency.

After I told the woman we would need to hospitalize her kitten, she turned to go back to an empty house. I carried the kitten toward the back treatment area. There was no trace of the playful, carefree kitten she must have been until the day before. All her facial muscles were strained and tight with the effort to keep breathing. This terror could leave a shadow upon her.

"Get the oxygen, guys!" I shouted, slamming through the door. Oxygen was a necessity because the kitten's tongue was turning blue, and I slipped her nose into the rubber opening of the mask. She breathed easier. What injections should I use? I hastily debated with myself. If I gave her a steroid injection, she would probably improve quickly—but then her suppressed immune system would affect the vaccine's efficacy. I thought she was too young for such strong medication. But I had just been to a seminar on treating acute emergencies with homeopathy and, I decided, this was a perfect time to put this form of holistic medicine to use. Steroids could be a last resort. I rummaged through my personal supply bag to find a small amber bottle marked "*Apis* 200C." I poured the pellets into the kitten's mouth and hurriedly placed her nose back into the oxygen mask.

Tanya and I watched, glancing at each other nervously, as the kitten breathed. Although I didn't mind Tanya knowing I had used homeopathy, I really didn't want the other more conventional vets to know how I was treating the kitten, because homeopathy was still considered "fringe medicine." After fifteen minutes, she was still lying on her side, breathing with difficulty. Her temperature was now a little lower, 104 Fahrenheit. There were so many other patients waiting that I had to put Pounces in a cage and go to my next exam room. Tanya was to take her temperature every ten minutes.

It seemed like just minutes, but over an hour had gone by when Tanya stopped me in the hallway. "That kitten is up and walking around like nothing happened!" she exclaimed. I ran back to see her. She was standing in her cage, crunching her upper lip and whiskers in between the bars, as only cats do to show their happiness. She was breathing normally now; the terror was gone from her eyes.

I became angry at my profession's hand in causing Pounces's reaction, as well as the powerful vaccine-producing companies that feed our fear of infectious organisms to the point that, without any solid scientific evidence, we vaccinate our pets annually. Were the words of our veterinary oath, "Above all, do no harm," just empty sentiment handed down by ancient physicians, or were they wise words not to be taken lightly? As I handed the purring kitten over to her human parent, the woman cried tears of relief that Pounces was alive. She waved goodbye, and the kitten took one last look at me before the two vanished from my sight.

As I entered the doctor's office to write up records, I looked up at my picture of Smudge on the beach. In the early morning hours, after a busy night, I began to see that I needed to discover another way to treat animals. As I said goodbye to Tanya, that morning I also bid farewell to animal ER: the surgeries, lacerations, and abscesses. ER veterinarians have a tough job, especially given that they're paid about one fourth of human doctors' salaries. I'm comforted to know there are great conventional veterinarians helping animals at night as well as in the daytime. Although I believe there are serious problems with vaccines and with certain long-term medications, I know most veterinarians are trying their best and working from their hearts.

I drove home, smuggling the cute little white boxer puppy with me. Snug in a towel on my lap, he suckled on my finger, pretending I was his mother. In two days, when his littermates would be getting their tails snipped off without anesthesia to maintain breed standards, this little puppy would be with a technician friend who saves white boxers. In a few weeks, when his siblings would be getting their ears cropped, he would be adopted by new parents, and, with tail and ears unharmed, he would be able to communicate his emotions with an intact body. When he was sad, he would still be able to tuck his tail under and lower his ears. When he was overjoyed to see his new parents, he'd wag his tail and prick up his ears with happiness, I imagined.

It occurred to me then that I was on my way to finding a compassionate way to heal animals. I decided to practice holistic veterinary medicine. Although it meant more school, plane trips, and studying, I had to find a way to practice from my heart. For a moment, as I drove to drop off the puppy, I picked up the pace just like horses do when they know they are on the way home.

Emergency Basics

The following tables are meant to be a guide to acute symptoms and are **not meant to replace veterinary care.** Any medicine with a number and letter together after the name (such as 30C or 6X—referring to the dilution and strength) is homeopathic. Homeopathy is a form of holistic medicine that energetically shifts the body to become more normal by providing a medicine that in large amounts might cause the same symptoms that minuscule, dilute doses can cure. The dose is the same regardless of the size of the patient, about 3 to 5 pellets by mouth. Use a remedy such as *Phosphorus* 30C more frequently, say every ten minutes, for bleeding, and a remedy such as *Arnica* 30C less often, say three times a day, for limping. Mild diarrhea could be treated with *Nux vomica* 30C every other day, because the symptom is less serious. These remedies can be given alongside conventional vetcrinary care. Give all homeopathic medicines on a limited basis—for only two or three days—not because they will be harmful but rather because they will cease to be helpful if overused. Do not touch homeopathic pellets or drops directly, as this can interfere with their energetic properties. Do not give them with food. Give them on an empty stomach if possible. Place the pellets in a spoon with water, lift the upper lip at the corner of the mouth, and place the liquid in the pocket between the teeth and lip; or insert the pellets directly into the mouth. All homeopathic remedies listed below are readily available from health food stores and internet suppliers, or through specialty mail order (see Resources, page 263).

CATS

If cat owners kept their feline friends *inside,* especially during cold weather, veterinarians might have less to do. Indeed, most feline emergencies are related to outdoor activities such as getting into toxins (antifreeze), abscesses from cat fights, trauma from cars or garage doors, and viral diseases. Many other accidents happen as cats try to get warm in the winter; they include getting caught in car fan belts or laundry dryers. For all suburban folks, what about training your cat to go on a harness for supervised walks?

Other common emergencies include intestinal foreign-body obstructions from eating the wrong things. Linear foreign bodies such as yarn, ribbon, and thread—sewing needles are especially dangerous when there is a thread attached—can act like a sharp knife in the intestines and can cause damage that requires surgery. Trouble breathing or other respiratory distress may result from chest fluid due to heart problems, asthma, or cancer. Do not give cats acetaminophen (Tylenol), ibuprofen, or large doses of aspirin (even 325 milligrams), because cats lack the enzyme glutathione peroxidase, which helps break down these anti-inflammatory medications.

CAT SYMPTOMS	POSSIBLE CAUSES	YOUR ACTION
Bleeding from nose, mouth, or skin	Trauma, liver disease, rodent poison from eating a poisoned mouse or rat	Apply direct pressure; GO TO VET. *Phosphorus* 30C, Yunnan Pai Yao[1]
Puncture of skin	Cat bite, sharp object	Clean wound with antimicrobial solution/ Epsom salts and warm water[2]; GO TO VET. *Silicea* 30C, *Ledum* 30C

1. Give ½ capsule (cover the open end with butter to avoid spilling the powder) for a 10- to 15-pound cat; repeat up to 3 times a day. This is a safe Chinese herbal formula.
2. Mix 1 teaspoon Epsom salts and ½ teaspoon povidine antibiotic solution per cup warm water. Povidine is an iodine-based antibiotic solution available in a drugstore. It is not to be used if your pet is allergic to iodine.

CAT SYMPTOMS	POSSIBLE CAUSES	YOUR ACTION
Limping	Soft tissue injury, fracture, dislocation of joint	If weight bearing, *Arnica* 30C; if non-weight-bearing[3] or not improving within 24 hours, GO TO VET.
Unable to move hind legs	Saddle thrombus (blood clot), trauma to spine/pelvis	GO TO VET.
Straining to urinate	Male: blocked urination or cystitis. Female: bladder infection or sterile cystitis.	Male: GO TO VET. Female: *Cantharis* 30C. GO TO VET for urine tests.
Constipation	Does not like kitty litter. Diet, oils, fiber, or water intake may be a problem.	1 teaspoon canned pumpkin with ½ teaspoon fish oil, moistened oat bran, or psyllium or Laxatone.[4] If more than 2 days, GO TO VET.

3. Non-weight-bearing refers to a condition in which the animal is not putting any weight on a leg and is essentially holding it up off the ground. An animal can have a minor sprain and be non-weight-bearing just for a few minutes or hours, but any animal that is non-weight-bearing for longer than that may have a ligament rupture or fracture. Veterinary care is needed.

4. Laxatone is a safe, mineral oil–based supplement that cats will lick off their paws or perhaps even right from the tube. It is available at any pet store and can facilitate defecation, especially if the problem is hairball passage. There is also Petromalt, which acts similarly.

CAT SYMPTOMS	POSSIBLE CAUSES	YOUR ACTION
Vomiting/diarrhea	Hairball, foreign body, parasites, inflammatory bowel disease	Check under tongue for thread.[5] If vomiting infrequently, hold off food for 12 hours. If depressed,[6] GO TO VET.
Lethargy/not eating	Fever from abscess, antifreeze poisoning, hepatic lipidosis (fatty liver disease), other metabolic conditions	If not eating for more than 1 day, take to vet. Feel body for swelling or lump, take temperature with digital thermometer[7] (normal is 101 or so). GO TO VET. Fever: *Belladonna* 30C. Anorexia[8]: *Nux vomica* 30C.

5. Certain cats like to live life on the edge, swallowing thread, needles, and other foreign bodies. Since there are so many causes for vomiting, looking under the tongue for a piece of thread is an easy thing to do. For some reason, it can often be found wound around the base of the tongue. These "linear foreign bodies" are among the most dangerous because esophageal or intestinal laceration unfortunately often have very poor prognoses. Veterinary care and, especially, surgery surely will be needed. In general, cats vomit easily, and one or two times may indicate only a hairball or other normal event. Any more than twice in a row, or if the vomiting is repeated intermittently over days, or especially if the cat appears to act tired or abnormal, take him to the vet at once.

6. "Depressed" means that the cat acts tired or dull as compared to normal. "Lethargic" is a more severe state in which the cat is hard to rouse.

7. Digital thermometers are available at any pharmacy and are much safer than glass ones, which can break. It is easy to safely take a rectal temperature with a little olive oil on the end of the thermometer. Pass the tapered end in about an inch.

8. Anorexia simply means that the animal is not eating.

CAT SYMPTOMS	POSSIBLE CAUSES	YOUR ACTION
Twitching, falling over, collapse	Toxins such as pyrethrins; if salivating, organophosphate[9] or slug-bait poisoning; stroke, seizure, metabolic disease	GO TO VET; *Aconite* 30C
Known poison ingestion	Antifreeze, chewable canine Rimadyl, aspirin,[10] acetaminophen, ibuprofen, flea spray, car oil that has been licked off	Give hydrogen peroxide, 1 tablespoon by mouth, to induce vomiting. Call poison control: 800-548-2423. (This is the special animal number and costs $). GO TO VET ASAP.
Coughing, gurgling in chest, difficulty breathing	Fluid in pleural space or in lungs themselves; asthma, trauma, heart disease, thoracic cancer	GO TO VET.

9. Flea or insect products containing pyrethrins or organophosphates are especially dangerous to cats, whose first inclination is to lick off the spray, thus ingesting it. Because fleas live the majority of their lives off of the pet, in carpets, floors, sofas, and lawns, treating the animal directly with these products makes little sense unless you are using a more modern poison designed to kill the flea when it takes a blood meal. Examples are Advantage or Revolution, but because they are applied right behind the neck, the cat can ingest them as easily as the older full-body sprays.

10. Aspirin at the dose of half a baby aspirin (81 milligrams) daily or 1 baby aspirin every 2 days is usually safe for a cat, but anything over that may be toxic, as can be any other anti-inflammatory. If your cat might have swallowed even 1 teaspoon of antifreeze (ethylene glycol), he must be immediately rushed to a vet. Damage to the kidneys can be reversed only in the very early stages.

DOGS

Keep your dog out of traffic and garbage. Establish regular exercise, and get your pet spayed or neutered. A healthy diet (see homemade diets for dogs and cats, pages 28–30), ideally home prepared with plenty of antioxidants, will alleviate your pet's urge to scavenge. Common emergencies include trauma from being hit by cars; reproductive, respiratory, and gastrointestinal disorders like pancreatitis or bloat; back problems; pain; seizures; and poisonings. For unspayed females, pyometra or uterine infection is common.

"Garbage gut" is very frequent in dogs, especially around the holidays. Dogs often eat tinsel, chocolate, and even glass ornaments. Care should be taken not to leave pets alone with decorations. If the dog's attitude remains normal, mild inflammation may cause minor vomiting or diarrhea. If the dog seems depressed or vomiting continues, immediate veterinary attention is warranted. (Veterinarians often use the word "depressed" to mean that the animal acts tired or dull as compared to normal. This compares to "lethargic," which is a more severe state in which the animal is hard to rouse.) The most serious gastrointestinal condition is bloat (or GDV, gastric dilatation and volvulus), which may cause immediate death. In this disease of large, deep-chested dogs (Great Danes, standard poodles, or briards), the stomach fills with gas and twists, rendering the dog unable to vomit. Other normal-chested dogs get it too, often when a concurrent disease like cancer is present, and the stomach or abdomen gets very big and tight.

Although chocolate is not good for dogs, more have succumbed to other poisons or cars. One Hershey's kiss will not kill a dog. It takes 100 to 150 milligrams per kilogram body weight of chocolate to see any excitatory toxic effects. Medium or large dogs would have to eat semisweet or baking chocolate, which contains a lot more theobromine than milk chocolate.

The following chart is for acute problems. It is not meant to replace veterinary care, only to supplement it.

DOG SYMPTOMS	POSSIBLE CAUSES	YOUR ACTION
Vomiting/diarrhea	Minor: GI irritation, garbage gut, or parasitism. If ongoing: bloat; foreign body; viral infection, especially in young dogs; liver and kidney disease, especially in old dogs.	If symptoms are minor,[1] hold off food for 12 to 24 hours, then give bland diet[2] (rice or boiled potatoes/cottage cheese). If major: GO TO VET.
Hot spots[3]	Fleas or other parasites, allergies, wounds	Aloe vera gel or calendula salve, Wound-Healing Tea (see recipe, page 41), or even wet tea bag held on the spot

1. "Minor" means the dog vomits once in a while, say once every few weeks. "Major" or "ongoing" means the dog is continuously vomiting, sometimes five or more times in a row. Care is especially vital if the dog repeats vomiting for hours, because he will become dehydrated. Conventional veterinary care is necessary here.

2. A bland diet might be composed of 50 percent boiled chicken or low-fat cottage cheese and 50 percent overcooked brown or white rice or boiled white potato. The important part of a bland diet is to feed a very small amount, about ¼ cup for even a large dog, and wait for about two hours before offering more, even though your pet will surely want more right away. If all goes well after a few feedings of a bland diet, gradually replace the bland food with his or her normal food.

3. Anyone who has been around golden retrievers knows about "hot spots," specific areas on the skin where the dog obsessively licks, creating ugly red patches. In almost no time at all, these patches can feel as if they are on fire. Dogs with hot spots have a hard time relaxing. Apply Hot-Spot Relief Tea (see recipe, page 258). Alternatives to the homemade tea are: aloe vera gel from the real plant; calendula salve, available at any human health food store; or a moistened black tea bag, which has some astringent and cooling properties. Apply your choice of these to the skin for at least ten minutes. A topical cortisone spray from your vet may be necessary. Acute hot spots are different from "lick granulomas," which are less painful and more chronic. Lick granulomas are best treated with acupuncture.

DOG SYMPTOMS	POSSIBLE CAUSES	YOUR ACTION
Swollen face, hives	Bee or spider sting, other allergic reaction	Human Benadryl (diphenhydramine), 25 milligrams per 40 pounds of dog. If trouble breathing or severe swelling: GO TO VET.
Respiratory distress, coughing	Trauma, heart disease, cancer, pneumonia, toy caught in throat, kennel cough[4]	GO TO VET.
Known toxin ingestion	Rat bait—causes bleeding after a day or two; slug bait or poison mushrooms—causes seizures, twitching, elevated temperature	Poison control: 800-548-2423 (costs $). Give hydrogen peroxide, 1 tablespoon per 15 pounds body weight, by mouth to induce vomiting if poison is noncaustic[5] and not sharp. GO TO VET.

4. If your vet diagnoses "kennel cough" or bordetella, give your dog some human echinacea (300 milligrams per 40 pounds of body weight, once a day for 10 days), or even better is pau d'arco in the same dose. These are safe ways to help strengthen the immune system. You can also give General Immune-Booster Herbal Tea (page 173).

5. A caustic poison is one that burns or ulcerates the esophagus when swallowed. Likewise, broken glass or some other sharp object can damage the esophagus. Since the esophagus heals with lots of stricture and tight scarring, damage to it can be life-threatening. It is not wise to make a dog vomit up something that could damage the esophagus.

DOG SYMPTOMS	POSSIBLE CAUSES	YOUR ACTION
Back or other body pain	Trauma, disc herniation, fracture, cancer. A common age for cancer seems to be around ten years old.	GO TO VET. Rescue remedy, *Ruta* 6C, *Arnica* 30C; buffered aspirin, 325 milligrams per 60 pounds of body weight. Do not give dogs any other medication without consulting vet.
Laceration of skin	Dogfight, trauma	If small, clean with soap and water, bandage (not too tight); GO TO VET. *Arnica* 30C.
Anorexia, lethargy	Infection, high fever, metabolic condition	Take temperature rectally with digital thermometer (normal is 101–102°F). Fever: *Belladonna* 30C. Anorexia: *Nux vomica* 30C. GO TO VET.

An Easy Cat Diet

This makes one day's serving for any normal adult cat. Offer the food for fifteen minutes twice a day and refrigerate between meals. It will last up to five days in the refrigerator. If all goes well, you can make several servings at once and freeze the food, adding supplements daily.

While dogs love health food, cats would rather eat junk food. They need to go to Fat Addicts Anonymous, because they love commercial pet foods coated with poor-quality fats. Ideally, of course, cats should eat mice, but only country cats are so lucky. Eating a mouse is a natural way to get vegetables (inside the mouse intestines) and non-factory-farmed meat, and it brushes cats' teeth, all in one meal! Many of the diseases in cats tend toward Dampness. This is why I do not recommend dairy products for them. Be persistent with the diet—try freezing it or mushing it up. For cats, food is all about texture, smell, and consistency. The most successful conversion to homemade food comes from replacing one kibble at a time with the homemade food. This slow conversion might take a month, but cats seem not to notice the change if you do it this way.

⅓ cup ground beef or chicken, parboiled
½ hard-boiled egg or ¼ cup firm raw tofu or cooked fish
3 tablespoons pureed peas, sweet potatoes, cantaloupe, squash, or
    asparagus (try vegetable baby foods for human babies)
2 tablespoons overcooked millet, brown rice, quinoa, or couscous
2 tablespoons ground raw turkey or chicken necks (a natural source
    of glucosamine)
250 milligrams taurine
200 milligrams calcium citrate (with magnesium and vitamin D)

As soon as you are sure there is no diarrhea, add supplements one by one:

Supplements
½ teaspoon nutritional yeast flakes (Cats love them!)
2–3 canned sardines a week (for omega fatty acids)
30 milligrams coenzyme Q_{10} (especially if cat has inflamed gums,
    which is very common)

pinch Icelandic kelp
pinch alfalfa powder
50 IU vitamin E drops every other day
¼ teaspoon cod liver oil for vitamin A every other day

An Easy Dog Diet

This is the basic diet and will provide one daily serving for a normal fifty-pound dog over two years old. Like your food, this mix will last in the refrigerator for only five days before going bad. You can freeze the food—but not the supplements—into small containers and open as needed.

1 cup organic, free-range or cage-free chicken, turkey, or beef, parboiled
1 cup overcooked brown rice or baked or boiled potato or yam
1 cup raw vegetables, minced in your food processor (broccoli, carrots, beets, etc.)
1 hard-boiled egg or ¼ cup raw, firm tofu
¼ cup cottage cheese (2–4% milkfat), goat's milk yogurt, or 700 milligrams calcium citrate (with magnesium and vitamin D)

As always, change the food over bit by bit, slowly phasing out the commercial pet food and biscuits. After a few weeks, if there is no sign of diarrhea, start adding supplements one at a time. Many of these supplements help prevent chronic disease, such as cancer, and are thus very important!

Supplements
1½ teaspoons nutritional yeast flakes (or other B vitamin source)
1 teaspoon fish oil or one canned sardine three times a week (omega fatty acids)
1 teaspoon cod liver oil every other day
90 milligrams coenzyme Q_{10} (especially if your dog suffers from gingivitis)
⅛ teaspoon Icelandic kelp powder (trace minerals; helps thyroid function)
⅛ teaspoon alfalfa powder (should be vibrant green color; for enzymatic activity)

100 IU vitamin E drops (or use ¼ of a pierced 400 IU gel capsule)
500 milligrams taurine (an amino acid important for cardiac function)

How do you keep teeth clean? You brush them, and, when your dog's
intestinal tract becomes strong enough after a few months on this diet,
give him a raw, frozen beef knuckle or soup bone one or two times a week
or a raw chicken neck every other day. In the case of a beef bone, leave the
bone with your dog for just a few minutes the first few times until you are
sure he will not be so excited he will swallow it whole! Bones pose a danger only because dogs get so excited they don't think straight. The danger
of giving femur bones is that the overzealous dog can get his jaw caught
inside the marrow cavity. I have had to anesthetize dogs to pry bones off
their snouts. Most undignified.

THE BIRD WITH BUMBLEFOOT

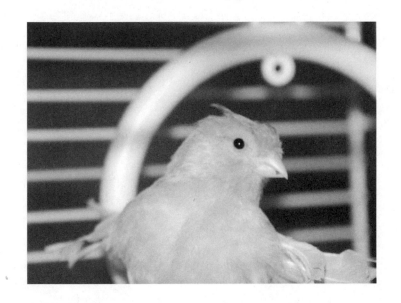

Many of the drugs we use for animals today were originally derived from plants, but in veterinary school I learned that plants are often toxic to animals. We students were taught to fear many of nature's most medicinal herbs as if they were pathogens, and to place our trust in pharmaceutical drugs instead. By the time I graduated from veterinary school, amoxicillin (an antibiotic) and prednisone (a steroid) felt as safe and comfortable to me as an old pair of slippers, while lobelia (Indian tobacco), equisetum (horsetail), or even St. John's wort were cause for great suspicion.

Gradually, I began to question this distrust of plants. At the same time, I saw that the very drugs I had learned were relatively safe actually harmed and even killed the animals I tried to help. More and more as the years passed, I opened up to the ancient art of healing with living medicine. I remembered how my French grandmother, Evelyn, used woolly-leafed mullein or gel-filled aloe to cure our sore throats or scraped knees. Her medicine cabinet extended to the plants perched precariously on the kitchen windowsill. My grandmother even preferred chewing pine pitch rather than gum.

Besides my grandmother, my first real teacher of herbal medicine (aside from books) was an unlikely little character, a frail canary nicknamed Chirpy. This canary could not sing, but his feeble chirps told those who were listening, "I haven't given up, not yet." Nicknamed Chirpy by the staff at the Bird and Exotic Clinic in Seattle, he sat at the bottom of his cage, unable to perch or even walk normally because of the large red callous knobs enveloping his feet.

For two years, my colleague Dr. Tracy Bennett, an experienced and capable bird vet, struggled with the treatment of Chirpy's foot infection, otherwise known as bumblefoot. This condition is thought to be caused by a bacterial infection, a weakened immune system, and a perch that is too round instead of one that is bumpy, like a natural tree branch. Tracy put him on a healthy diet of fruit, vegetables, and pellets instead of seeds. She tried antibiotic injections, oral antibiotics, soaking his feet in antibiotics, and changing the perch. Nothing worked. Chirpy's bumblefoot got worse.

"Just put him to sleep," the elderly lady who owned the canary sighed. She had given up on ever hearing his song again. "We've tried everything and I have my own health problems too." An unsettled quiet fell over the exam room while Tracy grasped at veterinary straws. Chirpy followed the conversation, moving his frail head from side to side, but his eyes focused mainly on Tracy. She had reached the end of what conventional medicine had to offer.

"Let me take him," Tracy suggested. "If we fix him, I'll find a home for him." They both looked at the bird, who seemed to realize his fate was being discussed. His feet curled inward while the large gnarls tipped him unsteadily forward and back. Chirpy's fluffed feathers were as dull as stone-ground mustard.

As a last resort, Tracy asked me what holistic medicine could do for the little bird. Gently scooping him off the bottom of the cage, Tracy spread his feet carefully between her fingers. The swollen bumps were red and hot. He squawked faintly in protest. His condition looked grim.

My thoughts traveled down two different roads as I compared the conventional approach with the holistic approach I had recently been studying. I decided not to focus so much on the bacteria and instead to concentrate on making the skin itself healthier. After all, it is normal for *Staphylococcus* bacteria to be all over birds' feet without causing disease. I could think of no better way to heal living tissue than by using living medicine. I went home and sprawled out with all my texts about treating people with herbs, intent on transferring that information to Chirpy.

Treating birds poses a special problem. Because their metabolic rate is about twenty times that of a dog or a human, drugs have little time to act on them. Most conventional drugs don't work for birds, and they may harm or even kill them. The more I thought about it, the clearer it seemed to me that with birds, safe medicinal herbs should be a treatment of first, not last, resort.

"He'll be our experimental canary," I said. We had nothing to lose. I made a list on a little piece of scratch paper of useful herbs for skin conditions, and headed for the only herb shop I knew, Tenzing Momo, in the

Pike Place market. As I walked into the store, under old wooden beams cluttered with hanging chimes and crystals, I was still practicing how to pronounce the herbs. "Cal-en-du-la," I muttered. I imagined that the waves of sandalwood incense were the hands of Hindu spirits guiding me into an ancient healing cave.

Large jars containing dry bulk herbs were stacked high to the ceiling. Their names seemed so exotic, and they were in fact from every continent in the world. I read the unfamiliar names: cat's claw, shepherd's purse, and yucca. *How did they come up with those names?*

The counter was cluttered with rings, stones, incense holders in the shapes of elephants and foreign gods. The herbalist scooped the plant medicines into paper bags, and when I hesitated, glancing at my list, he asked, "So what are you using these for?"

I stared at his nose ring. "A canary's infected feet," I uttered softly so no one would hear. I was not sure this herbal approach would work.

"Good luck getting him to cooperate. Let us know how it goes," he said. I hadn't thought about how we would administer this concoction but figured I'd worry about that later and drove home with the herbs in little paper bags next to me. I wondered what the real plants looked like.

Chirpy peered at me intently from the bottom of his cage, which sat on my kitchen table. I poured each bag of herbs into a large bubbling brew, and it occurred to me that I must look like a medicinal witch stirring my potion. Tiny petals of the golden calendula flowers fell delicately into the pot first. Then I added two herbs used by American Indians: the rich, dark-green leaves of plantain for relieving irritated skin and sticky grindelia flowers, or "gumweed," with their light, fresh scent, to treat the itch of poison ivy and poison oak.

I used other herbs too: the powerful antimicrobial goldenseal root, sage, aloe vera gel, and chamomile. The first addition to the concoction was the bitter-smelling goldenseal, which had been renamed by Samuel Thomson in the nineteenth century because he did not like the native name, yellow root. Sage, or salvia, from the Latin meaning "to heal," was added to cleanse bacteria, like so many other culinary herbs. The fresh gelatinous pulp of the aloe vera plant, or "kumari," the Ayurvedic name, would soothe Chirpy's sore feet. By the time the sweet chamomile flowers went into the steaming, whirling pot, it smelled as intoxicating as freshly cut clover on a dew-covered warm summer morning. The sweet scent eased my anxiety about trying this form of medicine; after all, Peter's mom made him chamomile tea to calm him down after he was chased out with the business end of the angry man's hoe in *The Tale of Peter Rabbit*.

Chirpy tried to sit up and supervise me. I worried about whether we were out of time, since it looked as if he hadn't eaten a thing all day. After brewing the concoction for an hour, I let it cool. I wondered how this brown, dirty, dishwaterlike tea would help the little canary who had been sick for so long. How would I apply the brew to his feet? Cotton balls? Spray bottle? No, I needed the herbs to be in contact with his feet for a longer period. I called Tracy and she suggested the "Tupperware route."

I poured some herbal tea in the bottom of a clear plastic container and placed the frail canary inside with the lid fitted on loosely. To my surprise, Chirpy stood calmly in the bottom and did not struggle. I placed the container on the counter, and Chirpy watched me closely through the sides as I did kitchen chores. He sat in the herbal brew for twenty minutes twice a day. He understood my tendency toward forgetfulness and occasionally chirped as if to say, "Don't forget me here."

Each day his head seemed to move faster and his eyes were more alert. He ate a little. On my days off, Tracy repeated the herbal soaks at the clinic. On the fifth morning she called me with an anxious tone in her voice. "Chirpy's feet are sloughing off!" she exclaimed. I had momentary visions of our toxicology professor's ominous face.

"What do you mean, 'sloughing'?"

"The big knobs are peeling off," she said. "It looks like healthy skin underneath." I rushed over to the clinic to see for myself. For the first time, Chirpy's eyes were bright, and he walked with determination over to his fresh vegetables. After eating his snack of broccoli and carrots, he flew up to his natural tree branch and perched proudly. I could finally see each tiny toe, although the skin was still red and raw. I couldn't believe my eyes. The big knobs were gone.

It seemed like a miracle until I realized that in nature, regular bathing in algae-laden rainwater would have been a daily event for Chirpy. He would have eaten a constant diet of fresh plants, and instead of perching all day, he would have been flying, as birds are supposed to do. All I had done was attempt to restore some of the bird's natural routine.

Healing plants and animals' immune systems are like old best friends. With intimate understanding and interdependency, the genetic material of animals and plants evolved in response to one another. Throughout history, animals have required the nutrition and restoration of plants, while plants have required animals to trim them and spread their seeds. The complex physiology of an animal enables it to break down and process each particle of a healing plant through enzymatic processes that evolved over millennia.

Yet much of Western medicine denies this ancient healing code and evolutionary history. We look for one or two active ingredients in an herb which, in actuality, contains hundreds of active ingredients that depend on one another to function. Only in the last fifty years have antibiotics, steroids, and other anti-inflammatories been in existence, and yet, today, they are used almost exclusively to treat animals.

Chirpy went on to full recovery in only seven days of herbal soaks. The little canary became my companion and his song greeted me every day. His bright yellow feathers gleam in the morning sunlight. Witnessing his rapid healing quickly shifted my thinking about medicine. His daily song was a constant reminder not to give up on even my sickest patients. My treatments would less frequently come from a pharmacy. In an herbal book, upon an acupuncture meridian, or perhaps, deep within the fixed joints of the spine, there would be a key—a cure for opening the natural healing vitality of the dogs, cats, horses, and other species that found me.

General Avian Care

Most pet birds are intelligent, active animals with great psychological needs. Birds are social creatures, and isolation or neglect can be almost as cruel as lack of food. Locate the cage near family activity. Be aware that birds, especially parrots, need over an hour a day of attention or they might scream or pull out their feathers in protest. Supervised flying in the home or flight cage may be beneficial, but not if the bird flies into large windows, ceiling fans, hot pans on the stove, sticky fly strips, or through open doors.

NUTRITION

A variety of foods are needed. The staple should be pelleted foods offered all the time. Organic Harrison's is available from your local avian veterinarian. Seeds are discouraged because of the high fat content and stress on the liver. *Cooked whole grains* should make up 40 percent of the daily food consumption, including brown rice, barley, and corn. *Fresh vegetables:* 20 percent of the diet. These provide essential phytochemicals, found in dark greens like collards, mustard greens, escarole, and parsley, as well as in carrots, yellow squash, sweet potatoes, beets, endive, and pumpkin. Avoid spinach and avocados. *Fresh fruit:* 10 to 20 percent of the diet including papaya, cantaloupe, and apricots. Most pet birds are from the tropics, where they feast on fruit regularly. *Protein:* 20 percent of the diet. Cooked beans or small amounts of cooked meat or eggs may be needed depending upon the type of bird. All fresh foods should be removed and replenished daily, as they will spoil. Milk products are not digested well. Calcium should be supplemented according to the recommendations of your avian veterinarian. (The statement "ABVP in avian medicine" indicates that the veterinarian has gone through the extensive process of being board certified.)

AVOID COOKING WITH TEFLON-COATED COOKWARE. Aerosolized Teflon has killed whole aviaries.

TEMPERATURE

A healthy bird can tolerate temperatures that are comfortable for people. In general, birds should stay warm—around 70 degrees is ideal. Sudden changes in temperature can make birds sick. If they are sick, one of the first things we do is warm them up to 85 to 90 degrees Fahrenheit.

HUMIDITY

Many birds benefit from occasional misting or having access to the bathroom while people shower. They can adapt to a wide range of humidity levels.

LIGHT AND FRESH AIR

It is vital that birds come in contact with fresh air and sunlight, as long as they are able to get in the shade if needed.

HABITAT

Housing should be as spacious as possible, as being caged can create many problems. Perches should be made from natural, pesticide-free wood branches from nontoxic trees such as northern hardwoods, citrus, eucalyptus, or Australian pine. A single well-placed perch may be adequate for agile climbers such as psittacines, because they tend to prefer the highest perch even if more are provided. Two perches, one on each end of the cage, should be available for finches or toucans, who prefer flying or jumping. Perches should not overcrowd the cage and should prevent the bird's tail from contacting food or water. Newspapers, paper towels, or other plain paper cage liners are better than wood chips, chopped corn cobs, or sand, in order that the number and consistency of droppings can be observed easily. Toys are needed, including a piece of corn on the cob or pomegranate, and small, nontoxic branches with leaves.

FOOD AND WATER BOWLS

Wide bowls rather than deep cups display food more attractively and may encourage the bird to eat new items. Placing the food at the opposite end of the cage from the water will help him exercise and not eat out of boredom. Clean bowls daily.

DETECTION AND PREVENTION OF ILLNESS

It is important to isolate and quarantine new birds, not from people but from other birds, for about six weeks to prevent the spread of disease. Being close to their wild state, birds like to hide illness, and it is common for them to eat and drink even if they are sick!

Prevention of Disease

Benebac or some other avian probiotic will help prevent intestinal *E. coli* infections. Certain strains of this bacteria are normal flora for people, living in our mouths and digestive tracts, but the bacteria can cause an infection in birds with immune systems weakened by human contact. Regular wing clipping and nail and beak trims are important, as are medical exams twice a year at your local avian veterinarian.

Evaluation of Droppings

Droppings can be an indicator of your bird's health and include three components. Normal droppings include a fecal component that can vary somewhat in color and consistency depending upon the diet, and urine, which is normally clear and increases with watery fruit or veggies. Urates are a creamy-white waste from the kidney. Abnormalities may include: decrease in number or volume, coloring of urate portion changing to yellow or green, increase in water content of fecal portion (diarrhea), increase in urine portion (polyuria), decrease in the feces volume with increased urates (polyurates), and the presence of blood. The owner should view several droppings in a day before becoming alarmed.

Other Symptoms of Illness

Broken, bent, picked, or chewed feathers; unusual or dull feather color; prolonged molt or continual presence of pinfeathers; stained feathers over nares, face, or vent; crusty material around nostrils; redness, swelling, or loss of feathers around eyes; flakiness on skin or beak; baldness or sores on bottom of feet; lameness or weight shifting; overgrowth of beak or nails; minor changes in talking, biting, or eating habits.

Symptoms of Serious Illness

Fluffed posture, decreased vocalization, change in breathing or abnormal respiratory sounds, change in weight, enlargement or swelling on the body, bleeding or injury, vomiting or regurgitation.

Wound-Healing Tea

Use topically for hot spots, chronic abrasions, or wounds that will not heal; for all animals.

3 quarts bottled or purified water
⅓ cup cut plantain leaf
⅓ cup cut comfrey leaf
⅓ cup packed calendula flowers (fresh is best)
⅓ cup chamomile flowers
⅓ cup packed yarrow flowers
2 tablespoons aloe vera gel (fresh is best)
2 tablespoons powdered Oregon grape or goldenseal root

Combine all of the ingredients in a large stainless steel or ceramic pot, cover, and simmer for 15 minutes. Remove from the heat, uncover, and let cool. Strain the tea, discarding the solids, and save it in the refrigerator. Apply to skin either as an herbal soak or with a cotton ball. Let tea stay in contact with the skin for at least 5 minutes twice a day. (Chirpy stayed in his herbal soaks for up to half an hour twice a day.) Leave tea on skin and do not rinse with water. It is safe to use this tea daily, but as soon as the affected area improves, you may discontinue.

Keeping: This tea will last for 3 weeks in the refrigerator if you are careful about not contaminating it with dirty spoons, etc. You can also freeze it in ice cube trays, and thaw as needed. If the skin is red and inflamed, it is best to warm up the tea to room temperature before applying.

CONTACT INFORMATION

Association of Avian Veterinarians. A list of avian specialists and a resource for information: www.aav.org
The Gabriel Foundation. A nonprofit Colorado rescue, rehabilitation, and adoption center for parrots: 877-923-1009; www.thegabrielfoundation.org

Foster Parrots. A rescue and adoption network that also attempts to curb
  sales of pet birds at large pet store chains interested more in profit
  than the birds' welfare: www.fosterparrots.com
Check my website for information about treating feather picking with
  herbs available from your veterinarian:
  www.wholepetvet.com/formulas.htm

COOKIE-CUTTER BAILEY

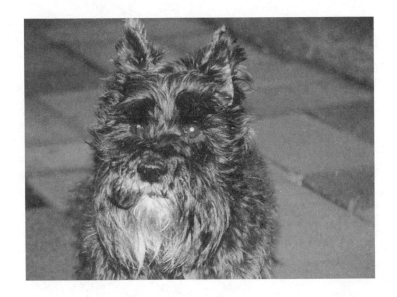

In the fall of 1990, at about the same time the Rangels added Bailey, an eight-week-old black miniature schnauzer puppy, to their household, I was just starting veterinary school. Little did I know that this small puppy would eventually teach me all that is wrong with vaccinations.

At the time, I knew of no controversy regarding vaccines. I thought they were solely beneficial. Back then, I'd just begun learning about the pathology infectious diseases cause in the body. I learned how effective a vaccination had been in controlling the infamous parvovirus, an infection that caused many dogs to shed their intestinal walls and die. Parvovirus left a lasting, memorable smell of terrible, putrid, bloody diarrhea on the conscience of veterinarians; the horror of seeing puppies die has fueled the pro-vaccine movement ever since. I thought nothing of vaccinating my own dogs; I lived in fear that they might catch any number of infectious viruses.

As the years went by and my training became more complete, I learned that keeping animals healthy was not as easy as merely vaccinating them. I learned that a strong immune system was the real key to health, and that many factors are important in maintaining the body's natural balance. Diet, stress, and emotional and genetic factors, as well as congenital immune system weakness, could be equally as debilitating as viruses, and these variables were much harder to identify than a causative organism.

In 1994, after graduating from veterinary school, I began working at a large ten-doctor practice near Chicago's O'Hare airport. I tried my hardest to fit in. Exam fees were ten dollars and were actually free with vaccines. Because our clients were good at sniffing out savings, they naturally opted for the vaccine option, usually preferring to skip the entire exam. Fresh out of school, I wanted to examine every pet from head to toe; this never went over well. The client would often tap a foot on the floor, look at his or her wristwatch if I went over five minutes, and say something like, "Hey, Doc, I really have other things to do." How could I blame the clients when our profession had trained them to think that vaccines were more important than a physical examination? I tried to explain to my boss, Doc Conner (we bonded over our common Irish heritage), that his policies overemphasized vaccines.

"What do I say when the clients ask why a pet needs vaccines every year but people don't?" I asked him once while he was in his element—the surgery room.

"Just tell 'em our immune systems are different," he answered, leaving me still racking my brain for a better answer. Doc Conner liked animals, but somewhere, maybe in the army, or in his thirty years of clinical practice, he had learned ways of preventing people from asking a lot of questions. I remember thinking, *I couldn't tell clients that.* Mammalian immune systems are more similar than they are different. The fact remains that even today there is still no medical evidence to support annual vaccinations. But not until Bailey arrived in my practice would I learn firsthand of the dark side of vaccination.

Before I met them, German and Debra Rangel had taken Bailey to several veterinarians and one internal medicine specialist for her immune-mediated disease. When this type of disease afflicts an animal, it attacks the animal's own body tissues. Bailey's immune system attacked her tear ducts, liver tissue, joints, skin, and red blood cells. Along with back and hip weakness, skin rashes, and dry eyes, the small schnauzer was also having more trouble holding her urine, waking German up to go outside in the middle of the night. They came into my office on a busy Saturday morning in November after reading an article about my holistic practice in *New Age Journal*. They seemed depressed. Having spent thousands of dollars on weekly blood tests, ultrasounds, and vet exams, the Rangels had become disillusioned with conventional medicine. Although immunosuppressive drugs had helped Bailey stabilize, she was still so weak that she had trouble standing up.

German described how Bailey got up in the morning. "To propel herself onto all four feet, she has to tilt her weight onto the back legs, lower her head, and rock forward," he said. I noticed Bailey's lowered ears and dull eyes. She seemed just as depressed as the Rangels.

"Oh, poor Bailey," I said. "She must have been very determined to get up!" I imagined her with her tongue lifted out of one side of her mouth, trying with all her might.

German held Bailey against his chest. German's black hair was pulled back in a ponytail, and behind his glasses his dark eyes showed the strength of his determination to help. Debra was quieter but equally distressed about Bailey's predicament. Neither wanted to take a seat when I offered it. This was their first visit to a holistic practitioner of any kind, and they weren't sure they wanted to become too comfortable.

Bailey too was uncomfortable. On my soft-covered exam table, she shifted her weight from one weak hind leg to the other. Wavy black locks covered her small body. Shirley Temple–like ringlets surrounded her shoulders and legs, while bushy black eyebrows enhanced her weary expression. German told me about all her symptoms.

"When was her last vaccine?" I asked.

German looked at Debra. "I guess it was just a week or so before the anemia problems started." A growing body of research shows that many immune-mediated diseases in animals are related to vaccinations. Vaccine reactions can occur weeks to months after immunizations, but the proximity of Bailey's life-threatening illness and her annual inoculations alerted me.

Being the superb clients that they are, the Rangels had done everything their veterinarian recommended, including getting annual vaccinations for Bailey. Every year, however, they noticed that Bailey became very sick afterward. She would throw up, become severely lethargic, and suffer from diarrhea. When they took her back to the veterinarian, the vet would give her an injection of cortisone and hospitalize her. The Rangels began to think this was normal procedure and did not wonder about its medical soundness until 1993. That year Bailey received two vaccines— one for rabies and one five-way combination for distemper and parvo— as well as her cortisone shot to prevent a reaction. But vaccines don't stimulate the production of antibodies as well when the immune system is suppressed with cortisone.

In the car on the way home from the vet's office, according to German, Bailey threw up and then became unconscious. She lay in the passenger seat next to him, her eyes wide open. He pulled over and yelled her name: "Bailey, Bailey, do you hear me?" No recognition. Panicked, German performed his version of CPR by blowing into her nose. After what seemed like hours, her head started bobbing, she blinked, and German turned the car right around. The vet admitted her for observation and then hospitalized her every year following her vaccinations.

Immune-mediated disease usually occurs in dogs who are well cared for, vaccinated regularly, and who visit the vet often, but not in dogs who rarely come in. This is a sad comment on conventional medicine. Perhaps in Bailey's case, her autoimmune hemolytic anemia (AIHA) was caused by the vaccines, which confused her immune system into thinking her own red blood cells were foreign. But whatever the cause, in immune-mediated disease the immune system *attacks* its own red blood cells; this is a disease common in cocker spaniels and terriers.

When I asked German to describe what happened to Bailey during her bouts of AIHA, the color drained from his dark features. "Bailey stopped walking on her own. Her gums and the skin on her ears, and everywhere else, turned yellow. She wouldn't eat or lift her head." He said that after several days on intravenous fluids and medication at the vet's, and after more prednisone pills at home, Bailey did improve. Predisone is a steroid that suppresses the immune system, and it prevented Bailey's system from destroying its own red blood cells. She wasn't anemic anymore, and was eating after conventional treatment, but her liver disease and her weak back legs did not improve. Debra fought back tears while the two gently stroked Bailey's lowered head.

"Bailey will be just fine," I reassured them, truly believing she would eventually recover. Her symptoms were straightforward and relatively easy to treat with acupuncture and herbs.

While I examined Bailey, I tried to explain the differences between the conventional approach and the Eastern, or holistic, way of treating Bailey's problems. "Sometimes conventional medicine is the way to go. It's great for emergencies and sometimes for surgery, but for long-term, deeply rooted, and escalating chronic disease, conventional medicine is fairly limited. It uses linear philosophy, which you, with your engineering backgrounds, probably understand well. This linear logic works for some diseases—for example, heart disease. If a valve in the heart is not functioning, very predictable events in the body will follow. Thus, drugs are very helpful for heart disease." Debra and German listened, but Bailey was bored and draped herself over German's arms.

I explained that in order to facilitate a logical, linear approach, conventional medicine had carved Bailey's body systems into separate pieces. If the body is like solid cookie dough, each body system can be separated out into an individual cookie. These separate systems include muscles and bones, heart and lungs, bladder and kidneys, stomach and intestines, skin and hair, the immune system, and the nervous system. According to Western medicine, these separate body systems may affect each other, but they are to be studied independently. Thus, a person with both a liver and a skin problem might see two separate specialists. But doesn't it follow that a diseased liver might not produce enough proteins to heal the skin?

According to the linear logic of conventional medicine, Bailey's musculoskeletal problem—that is, her inability to walk well—is treated separately from her dermatological condition, the red circular pustules on her skin. Her autoimmune condition may be related to elevated liver enzymes, but actual liver function may be considered a separate issue. While conventional medicine was often excellent at relieving her acute flare-ups, it might not have offered the best treatment for her chronic whole-body imbalance. The conventional "cookie cutter" model of medicine results in multiple medications, one for each separate condition, often prescribed by specialists who don't even communicate with one another.

I explained that Chinese medicine, on the other hand, links seemingly unrelated symptoms in an attempt to identify the underlying pattern of imbalance. I took Bailey's pulses along the inside of each back leg; they were faint and deficient, but they were also "wiry," vibrating as if the blood were popping up to my finger like a guitar string. Her tongue was pale and purplish and had a dry coating, while her eyes were itchy and inflamed. "I think it's a Blood and Liver deficiency," I said, "which led to Liver Stagnation and Heat. When the Liver becomes stagnant, the Spleen becomes deficient, and is said 'not to hold the Blood.' That would explain each and every symptom."

German was wide-eyed and open to this other medical philosophy but remained as serious as if he were already attending Bailey's funeral. "I just wish she could be comfortable," he said. We looked at Bailey, who was subdued. It was as if all German's guilt had begun to accumulate. "We also wish we had not cropped her ears. We didn't know it would cause her pain until it was too late." The Rangels had believed that they had been doing the right thing all along; it was only evident from Bailey's discomfort and failing health that they hadn't.

"It is no one's fault. Bailey's immune system is sensitive. In fact, if it weren't for your love and care, Bailey wouldn't even be alive today," I said.

Acupuncture is great for pain; at least we could start there. It seemed as though we needed to work on one problem at a time. Or at least that's how I presented it to the Rangels. Truly, the only way to help Bailey was to address the underlying cause of her problems: the Liver.

There is a classic triad between the Liver, the skin, and the eyes, and according to ancient Chinese medical thought, if the Liver is healthy, the skin and eyes improve too. Bailey's skin was red and itchy, with circular lesions appearing, especially along the inside of her back legs, where the Liver meridian courses. She had been diagnosed with "dry eye" disease as part of her immune-mediated syndrome. Her back legs were weak because the Liver was unable to supply the Blood needed to nourish the "Sinews," or tendons and ligaments. On Bailey's conventional blood tests, liver enzymes were sometimes elevated to thirteen times their normal levels, and her bile acids were in the hundreds, elevated at least five-fold. Even Bailey's digestive problems occurred because Liver, Blood, and Qi were stagnant.

Not being connoisseurs of Chinese medical philosophy, the Rangels hardly cared that my diagnosis was Blood and Liver deficiency. All they wanted was for Bailey to stop her painful whine. They wanted her to move her neck, lift her head, and act interested in what was going on around her. German wanted to take her on short walks again.

With Bailey's head tucked safely in the crook of German's elbow, I slipped my first acupuncture needle into a point called Liver 8, which is on the inside of each hind leg. This point connects to the internal organ, the liver, via the meridian and helps it directly. Spleen 10 was my next point, also on the inside of the back leg, which invigorates the Blood. I also treated other points around the hips on the Gallbladder meridian to help blood flow and calm pain through endorphin release.

I felt these points in deep crevasses along the surface of Bailey's small body, searching for areas of heat, cold, or tension. Like her whole body, most of the points were cold and deficient, so I used moxibustion, which is the burning of a deeply penetrating, special Chinese herb, *Artemesia vulgaris,* rolled into a cigar. Debra had indicated that Bailey's limping and stiffness worsened in damp weather, an unfortunate fact given that her home is Seattle, and I hoped to counter the cold Dampness with moxibustion, a long-lasting, penetrating warm treatment. Bailey relaxed some, though she didn't sit or lie down. Most dogs lie down and sleep during treatments. Bailey would not let herself be so vulnerable.

After the treatment, German gently lifted Bailey into their car; he called me two days later. He reported that she seemed happier, and had gotten up more easily. He confessed that Bailey was the first dog he'd ever cared for who had lived longer than six months. His farm family was truly unaware that dogs ever lived longer than that, since none had even reached its first birthday. They were hit by cars, succumbed to disease or rat poison, or were even shot by his dad! After such a rugged childhood, German vowed to do anything he could for Bailey. "It's no different from a parent having to pay for braces or college. I just have Bailey's medical bills." With her matching pink rhinestone collar and leash, Bailey was the princess of the Rangel house.

German told me about a dream he had of Bailey prancing on a snowdrift, something she had not done in years. During our rare winter storms, the long feathers on her paws would cake with snow. The snow would accumulate, and pretty soon Bailey's paws would be buried in big, thick snowballs that had to be chiseled away. Later, German confided that he thought these were just pipe dreams. When he woke, he checked to see whether Bailey could even make it out of bed. He confided that what he would miss most if Bailey were not around would be the gentle pitter-patter of her footsteps on the floors and the jangling of the tags on her collar. These sounds gave him a sense of well-being, like the Sunday morning clanking of his mother's cast-iron frying pan when he was a child.

For the first few weeks, German brought Bailey in twice weekly. He knew it would require some time to help her, since it had taken her years to get this sick. We started her on homemade food, including a small amount of beef, oats, beets, and kale; a bit of molasses; and weekly organic chicken liver to strengthen the Blood and Liver. Bailey also received calcium and other vitamin supplements.

I prescribed herbs, which German mixed into her food. Fortunately, it's relatively easy to treat the liver because it is the organ with the most capacity to regenerate. I prescribed a combination of Western, Ayurvedic, and Chinese herbs. I had German make a tea with dandelion, Oregon grape root, milk thistle, the Chinese herbs bupleurum and baical scullcap, and the Ayurvedic herb bhumy amalaki, all of which are bitter. Unfortunately for Bailey, bitter is the taste that benefits the Liver—German used chicken broth for flavor.

The leaves of dandelion, a plant people love to kill with herbicides, can actually help the liver clear chemical toxins from the diet. Oregon grape root contains the yellow compound berberine, a natural antibiotic like goldenseal. The antibiotic quality of Oregon grape would also help the secondary skin infection clear up, a faster course of treatment than waiting the several weeks it would take for Bailey's Liver to become healthy. Bupleurum is especially helpful for strengthening the Sinews; baical scullcap cleanses dirty liver cells; bhumy amalaki heals drug-induced liver damage. There have been hundreds of studies describing milk thistle's ability to help the body rebuild hepatocytes, or individual liver cells. Many herbs for the liver work best over a period of time, so I explained that Bailey would need to continue with herbal tea for several weeks.

During her twice-weekly appointments, I had time to catch up on Bailey's life and unique personality. The needles nestled for twenty minutes, activating each acupuncture point, and German, Debra, and I talked about the black schnauzer before us.

German described Bailey's puppyhood first. Housebreaking, with a child's playpen instead of a crate, was a breeze except once, when the couple caught their brand-new puppy squatting on their Oriental rug. They both yelled, "BAILEY, NO!" Like a deer caught in headlights, Bailey stopped and held it until the front door swung open. Out she went, never to poop in the house again. She won't lick, beg, or jump on people or furniture without being invited. German still talks about the utter shock he felt when Bailey actually listened to him in obedience class, even with no practice. He had never known dogs to listen as well as Bailey.

There was one notable exception to the jumping-on-furniture rule. For a dinner party, German made an attractive array of finely cut cheeses alternating with an assortment of crackers and olives, on their best serving plate. Since Bailey had never violated the furniture rule, German placed the tray on a fancy glass coffee table, and he, Debra, and the guests left the room for a few moments. Upon their return, they found Bailey with eyes frozen wide, her front legs splayed out on the slippery table and her hind legs doing the backward moonwalk to get down. Unlike most dogs, Bailey did not eat everything or mess up the spread. She had removed each sliver of cheese but not one cracker, with the care and precision of a ballet dancer. Had Bailey not been caught red-pawed, Debra would have assumed German had forgotten the cheese.

During our acupuncture sessions, I learned all the odd things about Bailey and discovered that German and Bailey have a very close relationship.

He feeds her and walks her, and the two take naps together on the couch, Bailey using German's chest as a pillow. She barks at pine cones motionless in the grass. If it's raining outside, she stands on three feet. If German uses an umbrella, Bailey will not pee, because umbrellas break her routine. Once the Rangels brought home a friend for Bailey, a sheepish cocker spaniel, but Bailey pouted in the far corner for two days until they returned the intruder. Bailey sleeps with outstretched front legs forming a pillow for her head and snores as loudly as a fat man, though she's only a small dog.

After five appointments, Bailey was much better. Her eyes were less irritated, she walked easily, and her pulses felt stronger. She developed a ritual, which has since made her famous at the clinic, of constant, excited, high-pitched barking as she enters, as if to announce her presence. But although Bailey was better, she was far from well. Even after I added vitamin B_{12} injections to her treatment, she still became tired after short walks, her liver enzymes were still elevated on blood tests, and she wouldn't play.

I studied the Liver and was reminded of the Dai Mai belt meridian, a very powerful, deep meridian that I could include in Bailey's treatments. I reread my notes on the Dai Mai: "Harmonizes Liver and Gallbladder. Good for cystitis, abdominal pain, weakness of lumbar region, headaches, general aches all over, if the legs are cold, numb, and weak. Hip pain if Liver Blood does not nourish joints. Dampness in skin, especially between back legs."

At first glance, it didn't seem possible that treating just two points on the body could help with all these symptoms, but then I remembered that this combination of points is particularly helpful in rebalancing the Liver and Spleen. In Chinese medicine, the Blood follows the Qi, so if the body's energy is not traveling down the back legs as it should, neither will the Blood. This explains why Bailey's back legs were so weak and why she still had joint pain. It was why she had trouble holding urine all night.

I wasn't sure if it was the acupuncture or the accumulation of herbs, but by the sixth treatment, Bailey began to improve rapidly. Just two months after her initial treatment, Bailey was able to jump up out of bed, go on walks without tiring, and hold her urine longer. If we waited more than three weeks between appointments, however, she still stiffened up after walks. So, for several more months, Bailey came in every three weeks. She still occasionally developed red rashes on the skin between her back legs (along the Liver meridian); she had occasional left ear infections; her liver enzymes and bile acids were better but not normal.

Now that the Liver was less toxic, I changed Bailey's herbs to a more warming formula, focusing more on the Spleen and its function of rebuilding muscle and supporting the immune system. One danger of using so many cool, bitter herbs is that over time, they can actually damage the Spleen (similar to the Western pancreas), interfere with digestion, and be catabolic to the body. This means that the body needs to put a lot of effort into warming the tissues that the herbs have cooled. Over time, the use of cold herbs can actually weaken body tissues.

When conventional blood tests indicated that Bailey's liver function had returned to normal, I discontinued the original herbal tea and prescribed Shu Gan Wan, or "Soothe Liver" pills, and added the nutritive, Spleen-protecting herbs alfalfa and gotu kola. I later changed herbs for the last time by prescribing Lithospermum 15, a formula commonly used for autoimmune conditions. This is the formula Bailey remains on today. As with the other herbs, the Rangels just mix it in with her food.

Today, four years after I began treating her, Bailey is twelve years old. Her skin has cleared up. She runs up hills. Her blood work is relatively normal. The Rangels have a dog who seems to become healthier as each year goes by, even though I see her less frequently. I do a treatment every two to three months, while Bailey stays on her herbs and homemade diet. Last winter, German gave me a picture showing Bailey in a baby sack fastened to his chest, as if he were a mother kangaroo. She was wearing two sweaters, and poking out through the bottom, I saw two hairy black paws caked with snowballs. There was a twinkle in her eye and in German's. Debra held both of them close.

What's in a Vaccine?

In 2650 B.C., the Chinese observed that people who recovered from smallpox were resistant to further attacks of this disease. They deliberately rubbed the scabs from infected people into infants' skin to infect them. Although some succumbed to infection, the overall rate of smallpox decreased, from 20 percent to 1 percent. In effect, this was the first "inoculation." This knowledge spread to western Europe.

The issue of vaccination for pets is in the middle of transition at the moment, and honestly, there are no hard-and-fast rules. More studies are being done all the time that show the risks of vaccinating (especially studies from Colorado State University, Cornell University, and the University of California at Davis). I think what is becoming painfully clear to veterinarians is that the concept of annual vaccinations was never backed up by scientific data and could probably be implicated in any disease in which the immune system becomes hyperactive and misdirected. These are often slowly accruing, discrete, chronic diseases—like arthritis, skin allergies, and, of course, autoimmune and immune-mediated diseases. Since our profession is in flux, **you are in control of your pet's health and need to make your own decisions regarding vaccines.**

Perhaps the most profound problem with repeated vaccinations is expressed in the holistic belief that they cause a weakness in the body that gets passed down from generation to generation. Some homeopathic practitioners see the damaging effect of vaccines as an energetic tainting of DNA, otherwise known as a chronic miasm. This is a specific disease predisposition grafted onto one's defense mechanism. For example, a dog might develop a wart in exactly the same location that her mother did. This genetic weakness is believed to have been caused by a specific illness or incident, including vaccine damage. Years ago, weak individuals died, and those genetic weaknesses caused by vaccines or illness were not passed down to offspring. But now, through medical advances, they are, and the result is a weakening population. So, what we blame on "bad genes" may be more what we do to make those genes bad.

DOGS

The most commonly administered vaccines include an "annual" DA_2LPPCv, or DA_2PP without leptospirosis and coronavirus, also known as the combination booster or shot, and a rabies vaccination every one to three years depending on local laws. What exactly causes an acute vaccine reaction is an inappropriate triggering of the immune system, sending the body into shock. From a conventional perspective, long-term vaccine reactions are harder to understand because they build up slowly and accumulate over time. Individual animals probably react to different components, but the "L" of the Lepto fraction is often not included because it causes a high rate of adverse reactions. Perhaps some reactions are caused by the adjuvant, an added chemical that facilitates absorption into the body. The more viral particles and chemicals a vaccine contains, the greater the risk of adverse reaction. For this reason, holistic veterinarians like to separate individual components as much as possible to prevent overloading the immune system.

Combination Vaccine

This is five or six modified pathogens in one booster shot for prevention of the following six diseases: distemper; adenovirus, or infectious canine hepatitis; leptospirosis; parvovirus; parainfluenza; coronavirus.

Perhaps the most important of these is for the distemper virus, because it can be airborne or caught by indirect contact and produces a serious disease. Parvovirus is also dangerous in young, weak puppies or immune-compromised adults but is spread by direct contact with contaminated feces. Rottweillers, Doberman pinschers, and Yorkshire terriers seem to be at particular risk. Dogs with immature, weak immune systems are most susceptible to developing an infection with any virus.

Kennel Cough (Infectious Canine Tracheobronchitis)

Several bacteria and viruses have been implicated in the hacking disease known as "kennel cough." These include parainfluenza, adenovirus$_2$, and bordetella. Usually, affected animals are young or stressed from being kenneled. Although the disease is not generally serious, it is highly contagious, and affected dogs can cough and gag continuously, as if there is something stuck in their throats. This is distressing to both clients and patients.

The intranasal vaccine for kennel cough elicits secretory or mucosal-surface antibodies as well as humoral and cell-mediated immunity. This means that the antibodies created from a nasal vaccine are specific to that area. Blood antibodies and white blood cells also get stimulated, but not as much. If you do choose to vaccinate for kennel cough, the intranasal vaccine is most effective because it enters the body the same way the kennel cough complex does.

Because there can be reactions to any vaccine, regardless of the route of administration, and since this is not generally a serious disease—dogs almost always recover fully—I don't recommend any kennel cough vaccines. There are several specialists who believe that because the vaccination is aimed at bordetella, a bacterium instead of a virus, the vaccine is particularly dangerous and has been implicated in various rheumatoid arthritis–like conditions. Even without vaccination, kennel cough goes away as soon as the dog's immune system strengthens to fight off infection. Stress and oxidative damage play important roles; vitamin therapy works wonders.

Rabies

Unlike any of the diseases listed above, rabies is a zoonotic disease—meaning it can pass between people and animals—and is fatal. It is rare in certain parts of the United States (West, Southwest) but common in others (Northeast, Midwest, South). The rabies vaccine is made from a "killed" virus with stronger than normal adjuvants that can act as a neuroantigen (a foreign substance creating a reaction in the nervous system). This means its side effects may be damaging, especially with yearly boosters, and it should be given only when necessary. Immunity after vaccination normally lasts for several years. Vaccination for rabies is required by law in most areas, but the required interval between inoculations varies depending on location. Ask your veterinarian what the requirements are in your area.

Lyme Disease

The Lyme disease vaccine may produce immune-complex arthritic reactions, which happens when big, bulky antibody/antigen complexes circulate around the body looking for a place to deposit. Sometimes they deposit in the kidney tubules and other times in the lining of the joints. In this latter case, it is called an arthritic or polyarthritic reaction if more than one joint is affected. The Lyme vaccine is not recommended in areas where the disease is rarely seen, like the West Coast or the Midwest. It is more common in the states of New England, near where it originated, in Lyme, Connecticut. Many holistic veterinarians believe that in dogs the vaccine can cause more problems than the disease. In humans that may not be the case.

My Recommendations

Whenever you are trying to make decisions as to whether to vaccinate your pet, you must weigh risk versus benefit. In other words, if your dog is young, say under three years old, vaccines might really benefit him. If he is older, especially if he is not well, the risks may outweigh the benefits. Other factors include travel history, exposure to wildlife, and, especially, contact with other dogs and parasites that may put your pet more at risk. Regular fecal examinations by your veterinarian will help rule out parasites.

The other factor to consider when you are trying to decide whether to vaccinate is the duration of the protective immunity. Whereas the kennel cough vaccine protects dogs for just a few months, depending upon the health of the animal and the strength of his immune system, the rabies and distemper vaccines often give years of protection.

Some holistic vets recommend only the rabies vaccine for many legal reasons, and others recommend distemper and parvovirus vaccines for young dogs, as these viruses can also produce severe disease. If you know your dog has a family history of severe vaccine reactions, immune-mediated diseases, cancer, or skin allergies, perhaps you will choose to minimize the risk and vaccinate only for rabies. It is smart to weigh the risks versus the benefits of vaccination. For example, you may live in an area where parvovirus is very common—perhaps vaccinating for just parvovirus every three years or asking your veterinarian to measure serum antibody titers is a good decision for you.

Ideally, each animal should be assessed individually and vaccinated for each organism individually. It costs extra for veterinarians to have these separated vaccines available, so you may have to request them.

For the average American house puppy who is not exposed to numerous sick puppies, I recommend:

At 10 weeks vaccinate for only parvovirus.
At 12 weeks vaccinate for only distemper.

If there have been no vaccine reactions:

At 14 weeks revaccinate for parvo.
At 16 weeks revaccinate for only distemper.
At 18–24 weeks vaccinate for rabies.

I do not recommend any additional vaccinations after that. I recommend no vaccines that contain leptospirosis. I do recommend whatever rabies vaccines are required by law, normally once every three years. I recommend antibody titers (page 61) only for older animals.

CATS

Cats have amazingly flexible spines, and because of that, I think they have stupendous energy flow and an almost magical ability to bounce back after illness. Sadly, this gets disrupted by what we do to them. Commercial pet foods, annual vaccinations, and the overuse of medications have interfered quite a bit with their powerful life force. The world record for the longest-lived cat is thirty-six years. Cats are not really old until they are twenty, in my opinion.

Indoor cats do not need vaccines if their environment is stable. Obviously, if you take in feral cats, you'll need to get the newcomers tested for feline leukemia, FIV, fleas, and intestinal parasites before bringing them into the house! Outdoor cats pose the major problem when considering vaccinations.

FVRCP

This is also known as the upper respiratory vaccine because it is a combination of two viral antigens, rhinotracheitis, or feline herpes, and calicivirus and panleukopenia, or feline distemper. Except for the panleukopenia part, this vaccine is a waste of time in older cats because rhinotracheitis, like all herpes viruses, tends to cause problems when there is a breach in the integrity of the immune system. Calicivirus poses a problem only in kittens. Like canine distemper, panleukopenia can be airborne and is very contagious in young cats.

I believe that the overuse of this vaccine, especially annually, bombards the delicately balanced immune system and plays a role in common chronic diseases such as sinusitis, asthma, and other respiratory ailments later in life. By vaccinating for respiratory infectious diseases, we create these other respiratory diseases. Perhaps the panleukopenia portion of this vaccine may promote inflammatory bowel disease, although to date that has not been proved.

Since the viruses contained in this vaccine are grown on renal tissue, this vaccination may cause cats to form antibodies against their own kidneys. Some research from Colorado State University shows that this vaccine can induce antibody formation against feline kidney tissue. This is especially disturbing considering the growing numbers of cats that develop kidney disease, particularly later in life.

FeLV

Feline leukemia virus is spread by nasal secretions, especially in young cats, but requires prolonged, intimate contact with infected cats. A simple blood test diagnoses this disease and is a good idea if you adopt a new cat. The vast majority of cats contract this virus when they are under five years of age. For cats older than five, the risks of vaccination outweigh the benefits, as the vaccine has been associated with malignant cancer at the injection site, and it produces variable protection.

FIV

Similar to HIV in people but not transferable to humans, this disease is very common in male cats who defend their territory, because it is spread from bites or other wounds. Cats that suffer a lot of abscesses from fighting should be tested regularly. An estimated 5 percent of outdoor cats are infected in this country, but the rate is much higher in other nations. If your kitty tests positive to either FeLV or FIV, it is very important to focus on building its immune system even if he or she has no symptoms. A simple blood test diagnoses this disease and is a good idea if you adopt a new cat. A new vaccine was just released, but its efficacy and saftey are in question at best.

FIP

Please do not vaccinate for this disease unless you have a cattery where your pets are caged and undergo stress or oxidative damage, the key factors that lead to a decreased immune system function and the development of this disease. Although oxidative damage is a natural part of cellular processes, feeding a high-quality diet, caring for the teeth, and keeping the liver strong by feeding plenty of antioxidants that repair free radical damage all keep the immune system operating at a high level. The FIP vaccine is reported to have caused many problems over the years, and many people argue that the benefits do not outweigh the risks, even for a cattery.

Rabies
Outdoor cats in contact with wild raccoons and skunks are most at risk. Check your state's requirements, but a booster every one to three years is usually all that is required.

My Recommendations
For indoor cats, or cats with minimal exposure, I don't recommend vaccines, but I highly recommend FIV and FeLV testing when you acquire your kitty. For outdoor cats, I recommend antioxidants (see diet, pages 28–29). If your cat comes from genetic lines with chronic disease (ask the breeder, if possible), you may choose to keep him or her current on only rabies vaccinations or use antibody titers (below). I do not recommend combo FVRCP, but I do recommend vitamins and immune-boosting herbs for the first several months of life. Do not vaccinate for leukemia (FeLV) unless your cat goes outside and is in direct contact with strays.

> 10 weeks: Feline distemper vaccine (panleukopenia part only) without the respiratory complex.
> 16–24 weeks: Rabies vaccine and every 1–3 years thereafter as required by law.

GENERAL RECOMMENDATIONS FOR CATS AND DOGS

Separate the Vaccines
It is so much healthier for the immune system to give vaccines separated by at least seven to ten days, ideally even three to four weeks apart, to allow it time to process each one separately and not get overwhelmed; this also decreases the incidence of acute or chronic vaccine reactions.

Antibody Titers
Antibody titers are the best way right now of determining whether your animal "needs" a vaccination. These are simple blood tests that check for antibodies to individual infectious agents like parvovirus and rabies. If there are enough antibodies, reflecting long-term immune memory, your pet is considered "protected" from the disease. However, remem-

ber that this is only measuring one branch of the immune system, namely, the serum, or humoral, immunity. Humoral immunity refers to antibody production, whereas cell-mediated immunity refers to the circulating white blood cells that eat up infectious agents. Thus, a low serum titer does not necessarily mean the animal is poorly protected. Antibody titers are the best available test to date.

Airline and Travel Requirements

Keeping rabies current is all that is required by airlines or for health certificates. If your local boarding kennel requires other vaccines, please talk to them about alternatives, or find someone to do home visits while you are away. Don't let kennels force you to vaccinate if you have an aged or ailing pet.

Keeping the immune system strong through homemade diets (pages 28–30), vitamins, love, and exercise is the number-one way to keep your pet healthy.

VACCINES OF THE FUTURE

According to Dr. Jim Everrman, one of my teachers at Washington State University, vaccines might be more effective if, instead of under the skin, they were given through the route the virus normally travels. Viruses that normally are transmitted via the fecal-oral route (like parvovirus) would be best prevented that way too, say through special dog biscuits, and those that spread through nasal secretions (like kennel cough or adenovirus), through nose and even ear drops. These vaccines of the future would be safer than those currently available. Vaccine manufacturers need academic and practitioner support, but perhaps the public has the strongest say regarding their pets.

YOGI'S PAIN IN THE NECK

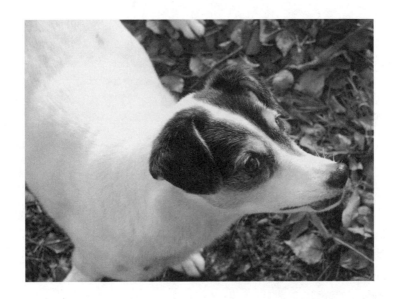

If you don't know Jack Russell terriers, you would swear they are too small to overcome what Yogi has suffered. But you shouldn't be fooled by his size: Like other Jack Russells, Yogi is small but scrappy. He is a little white dog with black and brown patches over both ears. When I met Yogi and Jim, in the spring of 1998, the six-year-old dog was paralyzed with neck and back pain. His formerly joy-filled, carefree life had become increasingly intolerable. Instead of chasing his ball or jumping on the furniture, all he could do was lie on his side, cry for help, and scramble with his front feet trying to get up.

After one month of treatment at a conventional veterinary clinic, Yogi's condition had only worsened. Every anti-inflammatory drug in the book could not reverse the fact that Yogi could barely move his head, much less his whole body. In fact, prolonged use of these medications had caused intestinal bleeding. Jim had exhausted all medical, noninvasive conventional options, and he was unable to pay for surgery. He came to me as a last resort and was, in fact, preparing himself for Yogi's euthanasia; he had even gone so far as to make an appointment to put Yogi to sleep. After all, Jim couldn't stand to see his little buddy in so much pain.

According to the other veterinarian, radiographs of Yogi's neck showed no abnormalities. Many people don't realize that radiographs can be normal when there is a disk herniation or other type of soft-tissue abnormality. Radiographs allow us to see primarily bone and large soft-tissue structures and are useful for ruling out fractures or bone-based tumors, but many spinal diseases, including most nerve or spinal cord abnormalities, may not appear on films. An MRI or myelogram is required to accurately diagnose a deep spinal cord problem. Many people do not have the financial means for an MRI, and myelograms can be dangerous because they involve injecting chemicals into the spinal fluid. Typically in veterinary medicine, people contact holistic veterinarians when the radiographs are normal but their dogs obviously exhibit back pain. At this point in my practice, veterinary chiropractic is a hands-on skill. With the degree of Yogi's pain and his trouble even walking, I felt trapped without an MRI or a spinal tap— it would have been nice to know for sure that Yogi had not ruptured a disk, developed a spinal tumor, or contracted meningitis. One thing was for sure, something had to be done. No matter what the radiograph showed, Yogi's neck was not normal.

Jim reminds me now of my words so many years ago. "I'll try to help, but I need you to promise me five visits." Holistic medicine often works best over time. Together, Jim and I gently lifted the frail canine onto my soft-padded exam table, careful to keep his body from folding or twisting. "Jim, do you know how this happened?" I asked, gently massaging the dog's rigid muscle spasms. Yogi let out a bone-chilling screech. I tried to soothe him by stroking his forehead, but his bloodshot eyes showed only pain and mistrust.

"No. Just found him this way after work four weeks ago." Worry lines deepened on Jim's brow. "He's been in a snail position for so long. It's hard to see him this way." He paused. "Well, a Plymouth Acclaim did hit him last year. Yogi entered right behind the front wheels, rolled under the car, and was spit out the back with the exhaust."

"What injuries did he suffer?" I asked. I'm constantly amazed by the stories of animal survival I hear from my clients.

"His pelvis was fractured, plus there were a lot of surface wounds. But he was fine after a few days. He could still walk and even run like before," Jim said, clearly still upset about the accident. "Hit by car" is one of the main causes of injuries we see in the emergency room.

"He could have back problems now because of that accident," I said, wondering if the immobile joints in Yogi's spine had worsened over the past year. Because it had been months since the source of trauma, at the very least I was reasonably certain we weren't dealing with an acute disk herniation. Yogi's conscious proprioception tests were normal. These are nerve tests that involve placing each paw top down on the table and releasing it to see if the animal is able to right it to the normal standing position, pad down. His other reflex tests were also normal. However, Yogi cried loudly enough that people two buildings away might have heard him.

"I'll be careful, but he could become worse," I said. I knew we had to try. At least Yogi was not a large dog with a big neck that weighed down the spine. I would be very cautious about the adjustments, basically attempting only to massage the bones back into place. The problem is that chiropractic abnormalities of the spine can be a direct cause of pain, or they can be secondary to other, deeper nerve problems, such as a disk herniation. The only way to tell without costly tests is just to jump off the deep end and fix what you feel chiropractically. If I did this and Yogi's condition worsened, we would know that his problems were too severe for chiropractic to help and that he would need surgery. If Yogi improved, his chiropractic problems were all that were to blame.

"Don't worry," I said, removing the small dog's collar—another common culprit that causes neck problems in dogs, because many owners inadvertently yank the collar. Over time, this type of repetitive motion on the delicate spine can cause severe chiropractic problems. "Yogi can tell you're upset, and that worries him more." Between Yogi's cries, I felt each vertebra in his spine and the muscles surrounding it. My fingers searched for the heat of inflammation or the cold of damaged nerves.

Starting with the "atlas," or the first vertebra in the neck, I moved the bones in every direction until I found the one with the most restriction— the frozen link in the chain, the third cervical vertebra, which had been pushed way out to the right side. This restriction, or subluxation, causes the bone to pinch spinal nerves that exit the spinal cord. I softly moved the bone and Yogi screamed momentarily, but after massage he sighed heavily. His eyes were still full of mistrust and misunderstanding, so I spoke to him without words, using only the language of intent: *You're going to get better, but you need to trust me and have patience.* Intent is a silent form of communication I had learned from other holistic practitioners.

Both Jim and his terrier relaxed. One by one I adjusted most of Yogi's vertebrae, but his muscles and ligaments still danced fitfully around my touch. While the chiropractic manipulations helped restore normal spinal movement, acupuncture would help control Yogi's muscle spasms and immediately ease his swelling and pain. Chiropractic treatment alone will alleviate soft-tissue pain, but when combined with acupuncture, the healing process is accelerated.

I gently threaded tiny acupuncture needles under the skin of his cold paws. He did not seem to notice as I applied needles to his back, neck, and feet, perhaps because his back pain was so intense. After only a few minutes, his eyes softened with the effects of acupuncture-induced painkillers, or endorphins. Yogi's taut facial muscles relaxed and he watched us sleepily. I surmised that the dog hadn't been comfortable enough in weeks to sleep. Finally, I could see just a hint of trust returning to his eyes.

About a year before Yogi arrived, since no veterinary college offered courses in chiropractic for animals, I had traveled five times to the unlikely town of Moline, Illinois, to learn the science of veterinary chiropractic. In 1997, the American Veterinary Chiropractic Association offered the only comprehensive program, although there were many short weekend courses. If four years of training is required for human chiropractic, how could it be possible to learn animal chiropractic adequately in a few days?

Amid the cornfields and the loud summer bugs of the Midwest, having followed in the footsteps of hundreds of veterinarians before me, I found my way to the classroom in Moline. In a large warehouse, surrounded by doctors from all over the world, I learned about the spine for twenty days, enough for the basics. Our teachers were both chiropractors and veterinarians, led by Dr. Sharon Willoughby, who had tackled both veterinary and chiropractic schools. I can still remember how confused I was listening to Sharon explain all the ways in which the first cervical vertebra can move. She blew away my previous understanding of the body!

I silently wondered why these chiropractors who had been trained on humans were allowed to touch animals at all. Gradually, like the other veterinarians, I changed my tune as I learned to appreciate the finely trained and sensitive touch of the skilled chiropractor. It required years, even after I was certified in animal chiropractic, to be able to feel small but vital changes along the spine. Since animal spines are altogether different from human spines, the chiropractors in our class needed to study animal anatomy. We had to exchange information and teach one another.

I had learned in Moline to let my fingers find the problems in a dog's spine, and I tried not to overanalyze. Holding up my plastic dog-spine model, I showed Jim the problems I found with his terrier. In Jim's words: "You cranked that model spine like a pretzel." Poor Yogi; his little spine was so crooked.

The rest of my prescription was for a homemade diet, antioxidant vitamins, glucosamine, and herbs—crampbark, corydalis root, meadowsweet, and marshmallow root—to relax muscles and ease pain. Crampbark helps relax muscles while strengthening the fascia, the connective tissue between the musculature. Corydalis root has been used for centuries for pain, and contains an active ingredient similar to morphine, although much less potent. Meadowsweet is an original source of aspirin, or salicylic acid. Marshmallow would soothe Yogi's intestinal mucosa, bleeding from ulcers caused by weeks of steroid injections and pills.

I was saddened to hear that because the regular veterinarian had advised Jim to isolate Yogi in a carrier, he had kept the lonely dog at the far end of the house. It is vital that a patient is not depressed or isolated while he is trying to heal. "I remember Yogi lit up when I went into his room," Jim acknowledged. While with a recent disk herniation it's beneficial for the patient to remain still, this many weeks later and so long after the injury, I believed keeping him caged now made little sense.

"Keep him as quiet as possible, but hold him close to you—on your lap. Massage his back," I said, showing Jim how to softly rub Yogi's knotted muscles.

Two days after the first visit, Jim called, cautiously elated. "He seems a little better. He's not crying as much, and he can walk again." I was surprised that there had been so much improvement so quickly.

"We need his muscles to be more relaxed for the next treatment," I said.

"Can I give him a beer? He always falls asleep after that," Jim joked with me. It was good to hear some levity in his tone.

The following week, there was considerable improvement in Yogi's condition. By the second week, his painful episodes were less intense, although he still cried when he was moved or touched. But following the second appointment, Yogi took a nosedive after chasing a squirrel. Jim would have been almost ready to give up if not for our agreement—five visits.

On the third appointment, Yogi's neck was arched again. He was unable to lift his head. It's hard to know what caused this relapse. Was his sudden burst of energy responsible for an additional injury? Or was his nervous system still in the transient process of "reshuffling," commonly known as a healing crisis? Some holistic practitioners believe this can occur when toxins and oxidative debris are slow to leave the body. I suspected and hoped that Yogi was simply experiencing a healing crisis, as he had improved so quickly following his first visit. If indeed Yogi had undergone a healing crisis, I needed to allow his energy core time to shift from the diseased state to a more normal condition. I kept the appointment short, prescribed more herbs, and told Jim to come back in just a few days.

Because he had improved at first, I was fairly confident that rather than deeper spinal cord pathology, Yogi had a long-standing spinal problem. I used electro-acupuncture after the fourth chiropractic adjustment. I did this to alleviate the stubborn muscle spasms that kept pulling his neck out of position. "I was a nonbeliever," Jim told me later. "I thought holistic medicine couldn't work. You hooked Yogi up to the shock box. It was unnerving to watch his neck twitch, like in a Frankenstein experiment." Electro-acupuncture is a treatment that involves placing electrodes on acupuncture needles, a painless treatment to reset neuromuscular endings where nerves and muscles communicate. It's especially beneficial when trying to restore energy flow through a meridian. In a case like Yogi's, the nerves are weakened or firing on muscles improperly. This nerve-muscle overstimulation results in spasms that only propagate meridian blockages. When I treated him, Yogi's eyes closed and he sank comfortably on the table, despite the fact that his neck was twitching away. Jim said he slept all night without a peep.

On the fifth visit, Yogi was almost cured. His third cervical vertebra was closely aligned with the rest of his spine. One common outcome of a healing crisis is that the patient will feel worse for a day or so, then improve by leaps and bounds. The redness in Yogi's eyes had dissipated; his pain had disappeared like a distant nightmare. I know that Yogi would have made a complete recovery with chiropractic adjustments alone; it just would have taken longer. Since Yogi's permanent recovery, I have seen many more dogs recover from severe neck pain like his.

Several years later, I still occasionally see Yogi to keep his back aligned. Without any hint of pain, the ten-year-old dog trots in wearing a halter instead of a collar, lifting his head proudly, and holding his tail high. He trusts me now, and that's all the thanks I need. Jim says people in the neighborhood call Yogi "Superdog." He really is able to jump hedges in a single bound. Jim calls the treatments on Yogi "miracle fixes," but I always tell him it's not miraculous, it's just chiropractic.

Veterinary Chiropractic

WHAT IS A CHIROPRACTIC PROBLEM?

In the olden days, a chiropractic problem was described as a "bone out of place," but now we refer to a chiropractic problem more specifically as a subluxation. Spinal subluxations cause swelling, which pinches nerves, compromises blood flow, and affects the immune system through impeded lymphatic drainage. Changes in nerve function, blood flow, and lymphatic drainage can also affect internal organs like the liver, kidneys, spleen, and intestines. Edema, or fluid swelling and inflammation, gathers around affected nerves, causing a vicious cycle that only pinches the nerves even more. This is why some animals experience relief with anti-inflammatory drugs. However, the underlying problem—the chiropractic subluxation—does not resolve with medication. Human chiropractors need training in animal chiropractic in order to work on animals, and the American Veterinary Chiropractic Association (www.avcadoctors.com) provides excellent training for doctors who want to adjust animal spines. Perhaps the best currently available training in animal chiropractic is through the Healing Oasis in Wisconsin (www.thehealingoasis.com). This two-hundred-hour comprehensive course is open to and taught by both veterinarians and chiropractors and is approved by the AVCA.

WHAT CAUSES CHIROPRACTIC PROBLEMS?

The four causes of subluxations are stress, trauma (even repetitive micro-trauma such as tugging on the leash or collar), toxins, and weak anatomy or conformational problems such as a long back or uneven posture. Over time, a vertebra moves a very small amount, but it is enough to alter the nerve input and output, blood supply, and lymphatic drainage. The biggest problem is edema, or swelling, around the nerve root on the spinal cord. This swelling temporarily goes away with anti-inflammatory medication, but the subluxation remains.

HOW TO USE CONVENTIONAL DIAGNOSTICS
TO TELL IF YOUR ANIMAL NEEDS CHIROPRACTIC

If there has been a recent trauma (within two weeks) and your pet is uncomfortable, go to your veterinarian. Conventional radiographs (sometimes called X rays) should be taken because back fractures, disk disease, or tumors are important to discover and treat with conventional medicine. An MRI is rapidly replacing the myelogram, but either may be helpful. A cerebral spinal fluid tap may be required to determine if there is severe pathology. Surgery, cortisone, or other anti-inflammatory drugs may also be needed in the short term. If all conventional medical tests cannot pinpoint a cause for back pain, or if you are worried about chronic use of anti-inflammatories, consider chiropractic. Symptoms from uncorrected chiropractic problems may go away temporarily, but recur, becoming worse with each episode.

WHEN CHIROPRACTIC CARE MAY BE INDICATED

- If the medical tests listed above do not explain your pet's pain or limp.
- As part of a preventive care or optimum health maintenance program, especially for pets known to have back problems (dachshunds, basset hounds, Welsh corgis). Use a harness to alleviate stress on the neck.
- If there is pain in the body that was initially mild and has become more pronounced, like a chronic back problem that recurs and, with every bout, may become progressively more painful.
- If you can see your pet is visibly crooked or has a head tilt.
- If your pet has one of the following signs: uneven gait, pain or discomfort anywhere in the body, trouble controlling urination or defecation, the development of an unexplained lick granuloma or constant habit of licking his feet (which can happen if your pet is feeling pins and needles).
- To maximize performance for a sport animal.
- For grouchy cats. Pain will make anyone lash out.

SOOTHE ME, SWEET RAIN

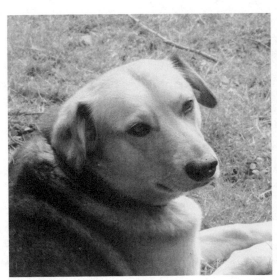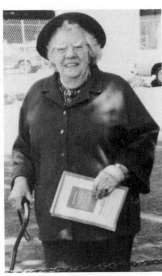

Breathing. It was all that was left. The familiar expanding and contracting, the hastened, involuntary motion of the dog's lungs was her only physical connection with her life. Ginger was a brown-and-black shepherd mix; she lay on her side in the animal emergency hospital, too weak to sit or stand. Her owners sat on the floor with her and I stood close by. They had hoped I would offer some last-minute miracle, but it was too late. We waited, hoping she would pass away on her own. The dog's chest softly heaved and lowered, her dark fading eyes watching us watching her. Fluorescent bulbs faintly buzzed above us and the minutes seemed like hours.

Ginger was only eight—too young to die. Over the past year, I had treated her liver disease using holistic medicine, acupuncture, and herbs, as well as conventional medicine. As the weeks turned to months, Ginger's liver became more diseased, she ate less, and her body weakened and grew thinner. The spark of life in her eyes faded. Western medicine had failed her. Holistic medicine had failed her. *I had failed her.*

I watched the last drops of fluids and pain-relieving medicine trickle through plastic tubing into an intravenous catheter in her front leg. The slow drip-drip rhythm fell in sync with the dog's fading breaths. As my thumb rolled down to clamp the IV bag off, I knew some part of me was also disconnecting in order to cope with my guilt and feeling of profound failure. Her owners, Claire, a single mother who was redheaded and clear-headed, and Emily, Claire's freckled ten-year-old daughter, sat on the floor holding Ginger while I functioned mechanically in my veterinary role. Claire braced herself against the wall and shifted to find comfort on the cold, white tiled floor and Emily leaned against her. They held Ginger tightly and wept tenderly. Love was all Claire and Emily could give to her now and the room vibrated with its force.

75

I well knew the rhythm of dying from all my years as a veterinarian. Ginger's dying was more shadowed for me—echoing my grandmother's death in the human hospital only three months earlier. Her IV bag also dripped and was eventually disconnected, her EKG faded, and her breathing was also replaced with stillness. All the color vanished, leaving only a stiff, open jaw, from which spirited, opinionated words had once been spoken.

Talking had always been my grandmother's special gift. In the 1960s she worked as a secretary on the eighteenth floor of the Interchurch Headquarters on Riverside Drive in New York City. The famous civil rights leaders Stokely Carmichael and H. Rap Brown had taken over several floors of the building, including hers, for a two-week period. Several church workers were expected to leave, but my grandmother stayed to talk to them. Since she ran Reformed Presbyterian Church caravans offering troubled inner-city children the chance to travel out west each summer, Carmichael regarded her as "a soul sister," and she continued to work alongside the United Black Front. Unlike many whites of that time, she was not afraid of Carmichael's call for black power and understood that his radical opinions arose from experiences in the segregated South—witnessing peaceful protesters being beaten, brutalized, and killed for seeking the ordinary rights of citizens.

"You must always try to listen when you do not agree with someone," she said one summer day years later while we shared a bowl of popcorn. "Everyone gets so attached to their opinion. Listen and think. I have learned some of life's most precious lessons by reflecting on arguments I had many years ago."

Gramma grew too old to properly care for herself and too proud to admit it. With her family living on the other side of the country, nobody noticed that she had slowly become weaker until her immune system failed her and she developed an infection. But her philosophy on life and death had helped me for years as a veterinarian in trying to help owners accept the loss of a pet. For my grandmother, each day truly was a gift, since she had almost died at age eighteen from spinal meningitis. Her faith was strong; and just as with the beloved dog beside us, I saw no fear in her eyes.

Secretly, Ginger was one of my favorite animal patients, and with all my heart, I wanted her to live, to thrive again. Her large brown eyes were bordered with dark lines, allowing her pure expression of emotion. Because it looked as if someone made her up every day, her owners and I called her

Maybelline Girl. She reminded me so much of Julieta, also a shepherd, possibly crossed with a platypus, since she was only a foot tall but four feet long. Julieta had helped me cope with the stresses of my childhood life— my parents' divorce, and moving, always moving.

Claire, Emily, and I lifted Ginger with a pink-and-green towel under her belly. I padded the floor beneath her with more towels while her family and I continued to say goodbye to her. Her head drooped weakly toward the floor, and all of her ribs were visible even through her thick undercoat. "She hasn't eaten in five days," Claire said, as if reading my mind about how thin the dog appeared. "We tried everything, even baby food and eggs, her favorite." Tears softly rolled down her cheeks. Emily stood awkwardly fiddling with her fingers, hidden behind her back, but after a few minutes sat down next to her dog, strangely peaceful. She wiped the sandy blond hair from her eyes and looked down at Ginger.

She bluntly said, "Ginger's going to die—huh?" and looked up at me in my white doctor's coat with a stethoscope snugly coiled around my neck.

"There's nothing more I can do for her. We have tried everything." I looked at both of them. I was trying to be brave and not allow the painful guilt to constrict my throat. "I'm so sorry," I finally uttered quietly.

Claire sighed and looked down at Ginger, who was breathing more heavily now. But Emily looked up at me again, touched my hand, and said, "It will be okay. Ginger will go keep Grandma company, right, Mom?" Emily had also lost a grandmother recently.

"Right," Claire said without hesitation, and seemed a little stronger from saying it. But I was less at peace than they were. What if Claire had gone to another holistic veterinarian, one with more years' experience? Was there something else I could have tried? My conventional veterinary training focused on the continuation of life, never the acceptance of death. We veterinary students were never given any guidance on how to help clients cope with the loss of their pets.

In lecture after lecture, hour after hour, our professors spoke of newer technology, updated diagnostic tests, and the need for more specialists. Death was not discussed; it was referred to in passing as a "medical failure." In my naiveté, I was swept away, armed with the latest advances in medicine; I hoped that I too could always save lives.

What veterinary training had denied me, my grandmother tried to instill within me—a great respect for spirituality and the acceptance of death. She attempted to teach me to honor that tired inner spirit instead of forcing it to occupy a body longer than necessary. Once, while we were chopping vegetables, my grandmother discussed her own wishes. Arthritis and a hunched spine rendered her too tired to stand, so she sat at the table while I stood with my back facing her.

"I want to die with my boots on," she boldly proclaimed while hunched over some onions. She had always blurted out her private feelings at strange times. "I don't want any heroics, and I'm not afraid of death. I've been lucky to live this long." She teared up a little but maybe it was the sting of the onions.

I said nothing, just turned and looked at her. She continued, "When your great-grandmother, my mother, was dying, Doc Hayes came to the farmhouse—doctors did that back then. He said she was filling up with water."

I was disgusted with such simplistic medical proclamations. After all, it was 1993; I was in my junior year at vet school. I had spent months learning how to diagnose heart conditions and interpret blood tests—albeit for animals. From my high horse, I said, "Gram, filling up with water can mean so many things. Was it her heart or kidneys or what?"

She retorted, "Well, I don't know. They didn't run tests back then, but what did it matter? Ma was over sixty and was ready to go." At the time I was horrified; how could they not try to save their own mother? Years later, I realized Gram was trying to show me how to accept the fact that yes, people, as well as animals, die. Death is always part of life no matter how many medical advances there are.

On the night Ginger came in, I wanted to flee the exam room where she lay breathing; I wanted to flee the hospital where so many other animals could not be saved. I wished some other critical emergency would be rushed in to get my mind off Ginger, but none was. When there was no hope of recovery for my grandmother, her doctors made themselves scarce, unavailable for our unanswered questions. So now, as hard as it was to be present for Claire and Emily, the urge to face the responsibility kept my feet stuck firmly to the hospital floor even though I was unsure of what to say or not say.

Ginger closed her tired eyes, and Claire sat, exhausted, cradling the dog's head in her hand, stroking her dry flaky fur. Rather than shielding Emily from the truth, Claire kept her daughter by her side. The child occasionally slept, or pretended to do so, on the hard cold floor beneath them. I sat down next to them.

After a long silence, Claire recounted every memorable event spent with Ginger. When they'd first picked her out at the pound seven years ago, they'd known she was the dog for them when she'd peed unabashedly on Claire's new black pumps. For a moment, we all giggled. In Ginger's happiness with simple things, like eating, walking, and being with her loved ones, Claire found the strength to do the same, even after a painful divorce. It was Ginger, Claire confided in me, who'd chosen the new house by planting herself in the center of the living room and folding her front paw firmly under her.

After the divorce, it was Ginger who'd broken the morose mood in the house. She did so cleverly. When Emily accidentally dropped a grape on the floor, Ginger seized the moment, taking the grape into her mouth and quickly, deliberately flicking it back out across the room. She barked and chased it all over the house, wagging her tail. Eventually Claire and Emily both laughed, even in this most difficult of times.

Two hours after her arrival at the hospital, Ginger began crying, whimpering as her spirit struggled to leave her. The pain was evident in her eyes and she weakly flopped her head now, trying to escape it. We all grew uneasy. "Claire, do you want me to do anything?" I said after pausing for a few seconds. "I think I should."

The high-pitched cries continued. Claire hesitated. "How long will it take her to go on her own?" she asked.

"This could go on for hours, but I could give her some more morphine or Valium, which might quiet her some."

After a short time looking at Emily, who was in a half-sleep state, Claire made up her mind. "No, go ahead and . . ." She turned to face me. Tears welling in her eyes gave her intent away. Nobody hoped more than I that Ginger would just pass away softly on her own. It would be so difficult to administer a lethal injection to such a wonderful being, and I worried that I might be too shaken, too attached, too emotional to do so. But I knew, as my grandmother had taught me, that death was inevitable and that I could at least add some dignity to Ginger's passing by helping her to go peacefully. I knelt down in front of her and picked up her head. Her eyes told me that she needed my help now.

I left the room and took with me the bottle of thick pink euthanasia solution, a pentobarbital-based preparation so strong that only a little more than one teaspoon would end Ginger's life. Every time I euthanized an animal, waves of nausea rose in my throat. I never knew if feeling sick was emotional, caused by stress, or perhaps just my physical sensitivity to the powerful deadly chemicals penetrating my skin. Guilt ate away at my stomach as I drew the solution for Ginger into a syringe.

I returned to the room and asked Claire if she had ever been present during euthanasia before and if she wanted Emily there. "This is the first time, but I want Emily here. Tell us what happens," she said softly, supporting her hand on Emily's leg.

"There are two chemicals in this pink solution. One that stops the brain and one that stops the breathing." I paused to regain my composure. "The one that stops the brain works fast, almost as soon as I give the shot, but the breathing might keep going for a little bit," I said.

"Does it hurt?" Claire asked, still stroking Ginger's muzzle. She unconsciously clutched wadded tissues in her sweaty palm.

"As long as the solution goes into the vein, she won't feel anything," I said, kneeling on the cold floor in front of Ginger. "Just tell me when you are ready."

She nodded. I turned to Emily and said softly, trying to be brave, "I want you to know Ginger will be going where she is healthy again. She is in pain now and after the shot she won't be. She'll be lifted away from us."

Emily turned to face me. "Will she be lifted up to heaven on the raindrops?" Puzzled, I looked at Claire.

Claire said, "After her grandmother's death, Emily dreamed that raindrops waited until we were all asleep and then quickly returned to the skies to fall again later. She dreamed they might be like little elevators, and that while she is sleeping she could shrink enough to squeeze onto one so she could go up to visit her grandmother."

I was deeply touched. "Well, my grandma also died not too long ago. Maybe Ginger will get to her next life by riding on a raindrop, and we can visit her there someday." I turned to explore the face of the child whose imagination had struck me. How odd it was that she was not afraid. I saw no resentment, no judgmental harshness. In the deep blue of her eyes, I saw serene acceptance, a peace so loving I relaxed a little and took a deep breath. Though she was just a child, her words and her tacit acceptance were as comforting as my grandmother's had been.

I held Ginger's big front paw, the one I had put acupuncture needles into over the past year, the one that had pawed Emily when she slept too late, the one that had clutched her rawhide bones and scratched at the door to get let out. The dog looked up at me. She knew what was happening and silently thanked me. Claire and Emily cried while I gave the injection, and my vision blurred with my own tears.

"Goodbye, Ginger," Emily whispered, but by then Ginger was already gone. Too tired to fight after many months of illness, she did not resist the effect of the chemicals flowing through her body. The breathing we had spent so many minutes watching ceased so fast that we all continued to look for it.

We all sat on the floor stroking Ginger's coat. Claire solemnly removed Ginger's collar and a lock of her fur. I broke the silence before leaving the room. "Ginger knew how much she was loved." Emily hugged me and we all said goodbye.

Rain fell lightly as I drove home in the morning and I thought of my profession's hand in death and of Emily's dream. In memories and spirit, Ginger would remain with everyone who had loved her. Through my grandmother's faith, a child's words, and my ability to relieve Ginger's suffering, I felt less guilt and fewer lingering questions about my abilities as a healer. I had come closer to accepting death and hoped I could help others do the same.

Recommended Resources on Pet Loss

The first thing to keep in mind as your pet nears the end of her or his life is that it is okay to feel sad, and even devastated. Anyone who feels animals are not worth this level of sorrow does not understand the sacredness of the human-pet bond. Animals give us what people cannot, unconditional love, and when we lose that love, we are left with a big hole in our hearts.

I think the most difficult part about pet loss is making decisions about medical care and/or euthanasia. After all, what right do we have to take our beloved pet's life? There is endless self-doubt and grief surrounding this subject. People always second-guess their decision, believing it to be too early or too late. It is so difficult. We are always looking for a sign, wishing a little voice could tell us what to do. Just know that you are not alone. Although we deal with euthanasia on a regular basis, even veterinarians agonize over when to let our own pets go.

Having dogs and cats who live such short lives can teach us so many of life's greatest spiritual lessons—one such lesson being that of loving so deeply and being forced to let go. This is an advanced lesson in Buddhism that we learn just by living with animals. Do not blame yourself. There is a greater spiritual force at work.

American popular culture does not prepare us well for aging or dying. Instead of embracing the close of life, we deny it. As our pet ages, we are reminded of our own mortality. It is important that owners don't euthanize their pets just because they are afraid to confront death. It is sad to lose a pet, but we learn so much from the experience that can prepare us for losing other loved ones. If your pet is not suffering, it's okay not to euthanize. After all, pets have their own spiritual agenda.

MAKING A DECISION

When your pet has a severe illness, ask yourself the following questions:

- What is my pet's quality of life? Many dogs and cats can't walk too well, but they still eat. If a pet stops eating for days despite veterinary care, he or she may be nearing the end. As long as he or she is not vomiting, ask your vet about cyproheptadine, which is a safe antihistamine and appetite stimulant. Try another appetite booster, the Ayurvedic herb gotu kola (one 300-milligram capsule per 20 pounds).
- Consult your veterinarian or a holistic veterinarian. What is the best possible scenario? Can your pet improve? Sometimes it is hard to see beyond the pain or beyond a severe seizure, but there is still hope for improvement. Discuss whether your pet is in pain. Is your pet withdrawing from you and his environment? Isolation is one main sign veterinarians look for.
- Both you and your family must be comfortable with what you decide.

ONCE YOU HAVE MADE THE DECISION

Often, euthanasia is easiest and best if your pet can be at home and you are present. It is difficult at the time, but later you may be more at ease knowing he did not suffer.

If you can't have the euthanasia performed at home, there are many things that can help ease your pet's anxiety.

- Request that your pet's euthanasia be done as the first or last appointment that day. This will avoid waiting and traffic with other pets and people.
- If your pet is at all anxious, ask your vet for a sedative pill to give your pet before you leave your house. Or ask your vet to give a sedative injection a few minutes before the euthanasia solution.
- Remember that you have the power to make decisions about your pet's death and might feel less guilt about those choices if all goes smoothly. You should never be denied if you ask to hold your pet while he is given the injection.

BOOKS

Moira Anderson, *Coping with Sorrow on the Loss of Your Pet*. Second ed. Loveland, Colo.: Alpine Publications, 1996.
  I like this book because it is really a great how-to source for coping, in addition to having stories of pet loss.
Eleanor Harris, *Pet Loss: A Spiritual Guide*. St. Paul, Minn.: Llewellyn Publications, 1997.
  My favorite part is "Using Ritual to Cope with Loss."
Gary Kowalski, *Goodbye, Friend: Healing Wisdom for Anyone Who Has Ever Lost a Pet*. Walpole, N.H.: Stillpoint Publishing, 1997.
  This book is a well-thought-out, compassionate guide.
Sogyal Rinpoche, *The Tibetan Book of Living and Dying*. Reprint ed. San Francisco: HarperSanFrancisco, 1994.
  An incredible book for dealing with dying in general. I find "Spiritual Help for the Dying," and particularly "phowa" practice, amazing guides.

WEBSITES

Books of Comfort on the Loss of Your Pet—Good resource for cemeteries, memorial items, audiotapes, books, etc.:
  www.superdog.com/petloss/bookloss.htm

Pet Loss Support Page—Ten tips for coping with pet loss:
   www.pet-loss.net
Rainbow Bridge—On-line chat room where people can receive support
   from others:
   www.primenet.com/~meggie/bridge.html

ORGANIZATIONS

DELTA SOCIETY
289 Perimeter Road East
Renton, WA 98055–1329
800-869-6898
www.deltasociety.org

Excellent resource for information and references on grief and pet loss.
   The Delta Society has a directory of counselors who specialize in pet
   loss. They offer brochures, videos, book lists, etc.

TWO BAD LEGS

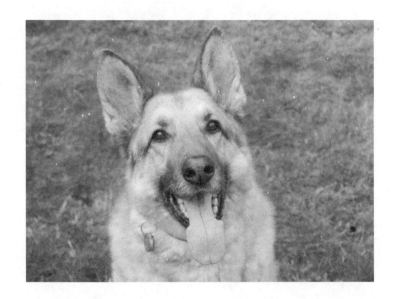

for a long time. *Films are sometimes deceiving,* I told myself, but the arthritis was so severe in so many joints, it was hard to remain positive. The left and right elbow joints, both hips, and even the spine were affected. The bones looked as though they'd been through a food grinder—it was hard to distinguish one from the other.

But I recalled that in many cases in my conventional practice, radiographs had not always reflected the entire clinical picture of animals. Sometimes dogs with terrible-looking arthritic hips could run normally and seemed quite unaffected by their condition, while in other cases, films of severely limping dogs were completely normal. I doubted that acupuncture was a powerful enough treatment to help Denali, but I reminded myself to treat the dog and not the radiographs. I told Andrea and Jerry to come in twice a week for just a few weeks.

Although the Sawyers were not the kind of people who would seek out alternative medicine, they were open to anything now. "If you would have told me to jump on one leg or stand upside down, I might have done it," Andrea later confided, and we joked about being so different from each other.

When I spent a summer with the well-known veterinary acupuncturist Dr. Allen Schoen in 1992, I saw many seventeen- and eighteen-year-old German shepherds in his practice. Not entirely convinced that acupuncture helped them, I spoke to some of the elderly dogs' owners to find out what their experiences had been. I listened to their stories of despair and of their utter surprise when Dr. Schoen was able to help their dogs. Shepherds are especially sensitive to the damaging effects of vaccines and can readily develop immune-mediated disease. Luckily, they are also very responsive to acupuncture. I remember thinking, as I returned home, that desperation erodes skepticism and success erases it altogether.

The German shepherd glanced at me with big brown droopy eyes, ears at half-mast. There are certain odd, unexplainable triggers that turn Denali from a cool, laid-back fellow into a dithering, panting, fraidy-dog. The list of frights includes a ringing telephone, fireworks, loud noises, and a three-pound Chihuahua that visits sometimes. But he was not afraid of my tiny acupuncture needles; in fact, he seemed to welcome the shift of his body from side to side to facilitate the treatment. Like other dogs in agony, he was ready for something, anything, to help him, and by focusing my intent, I managed to make him very comfortable as I slipped those needles beneath his thick brown coat.

What are the limits of holistic medicine? I always thought I had a good idea of what it could and could not do. In order to have success in treating animals holistically, I believed diseases had to be diagnosed early, before they became too severe. I considered advanced arthritis, degenerative back pain, and severe skin problems to be too difficult. I would not even attempt to treat cancer.

Then I met Denali, a dog whose will to improve was like a tidal wave drowning all the doubt about his recovery. I had misinterpreted his laid-back personality as a sign that he didn't care. How wrong I was on both counts, about him and about the limits of holistic medicine. Denali is a wise old soul in a very good disguise.

There is a sign with a snarling German shepherd peering down at you at the entrance to the Sawyers' driveway. It reads, "I can make it to the fence in two seconds. Can you?" If you're brave enough to proceed, you will see Denali, a large fluffy German shepherd who doesn't glare or even bark at you; he scans your pockets for treats or a rubber bone, his favorite toy. Whether you have them or not, he gazes up at you lovingly with big open brown eyes. If he really likes you, Denali will turn his head away from you, lift his tail, and sit all hundred pounds of himself squarely on your foot, turning from time to time to see your reaction.

One might confuse Denali's lackadaisical facade and his blasé sensibility with stupidity, as if he doesn't realize he's supposed to be a guard dog rather than a foot squasher. I got to know him and came to appreciate that what might seem like stupidity is kindness, and that what appears to be sluggishness in his demeanor is merely Denali's comment on the fact that the rest of us are uptight. His brown and black markings are flawless, his long coat soft and well groomed. On all four legs, he is daunting, debonair, and sophisticated—not the type to quarrel over petty matters, like lost bones or strangers on his land. Denali's favorite activity is chasing his best friend and female counterpart, Jenny, up and down their two-acre yard.

Denali and Jenny's humans are Jerry and Andrea Sawyer. When Jerry was a cruise ship captain, he met Andrea, who was from Switzerland, on the Mexico-to-Seattle route. Twenty years later, they are still married, and Jerry is now a cargo ship captain. In many ways, they are a typical American middle-aged couple.

The Sawyers are my polar opposite. They vote Republican. They eat meat (bacon and eggs is a favorite dish). They may have wondered about meditation and yoga but they've tried neither. Andrea smokes. Jerry wears a bright red Marlboro jacket he got as a gift from the company for selling cigarettes to his crew. Andrea collects knickknacks and is particularly proud of her unicorn and dragon collections. Although I've thought about having a collection of some type, unicorns and dragons would be low on my list. No, the Sawyers don't go in for holistic medicine themselves, so how did they find me?

When Denali was four years old, he could not walk without falling. His epileptic seizures were becoming more frequent, sometimes occurring every hour for three long days. Even more upsetting was the degree to which his severe elbow arthritis stole his happiness. Since Denali had been rescued, the Sawyers knew nothing about his history, but they did know he was rapidly losing his debonair dignity. His arthritis turned his young, smooth, round elbow joints into abnormally spiculated and roughened snowballs on the radiographs—indeed, the worst case I had ever seen.

Because of the pain in his elbow, Denali could not bear weight on his left front leg. Like many dogs who try their hardest to be good, he never cried out. When dogs are in unbearable pain, the sad reality is that they often don't utter a peep! We know they hurt because they stay still, act less interested in their surroundings, possibly eat less, and do not play. Denali would whine at night, unable to sleep, but most of the time, his discomfort was visible only in his glazed eyes. Just when the Sawyers were contemplating amputating the left front leg, Denali went down on one of his hind limbs, staggering like a drunken sailor. Now he was unable to use the left front and the right rear leg, and the remaining two were also weakening by the day.

The Sawyers had been to five separate veterinary clinics regarding Denali's continuing deterioration. The first one diagnosed severe arthri-

tis; the second one agreed but switched the seizure medication; the third one diagnosed probable degenerative myelopathy, a nerve disease similar to multiple sclerosis in people, which is common in shepherds. The third vet also recommended an MRI and possibly a nerve biopsy. But the Sawyers were wary of that approach, for although it might lead to a diagnosis, it also involved removing a piece of nerve, which might have worsened Denali's condition. Because degenerative myelopathy is a demyelinating disease, or one that destroys the myelin sheath around each nerve, it has a poor prognosis. Gold bead implantation offers some hope, but in general, holistic modalities are aimed at slowing down the demyelination with antioxidants and herbs.

In Denali's case, after trying various medications that didn't work, one veterinarian after the other had recommended the same thing for the four-year-old dog: euthanasia. When the Sawyers begged for another option, the last vet said, "Well, you could try acupuncture." But he also added, "It's probably too late."

What a shame, I thought when Andrea and Jerry Sawyer first carted in the hundred-pound patient on a Saturday afternoon. It was late for Denali, but despite our differences, I respected the Sawyers' stubborn attitude. Denali hobbled with his front and rear halves disconnected, like two uncoordinated toddlers. Because it would have taken him so long to walk down the hallway to my exam room, together the Sawyers carried him in. Andrea draped Denali's front legs over her arm as she braced herself under the front half of his large frame while Jerry cradled the dog's back legs against his chest.

I remember the surgeons in vet school discussing the canine gift of getting around on only three legs. "Dogs, after all, have three legs and a kickstand," they used to joke. But Denali had only two semifunctional legs and that was quite another matter. The handsome German shepherd was in trouble, and he knew it. His eyes were lowered to the floor; his grand presence was deflated. After a few seconds, his head dropped to the floor too. His canine knack for maintaining the will to thrive despite disease was waning, and soon his appetite might follow. I knew we had very little time.

I had spoken to Andrea on the phone earlier, but I still wasn't prepared for a patient in such pain. The Sawyers and I solemnly greeted one another, and I placed the radiographs they had brought in the brightly lit view box so we could look at them together. Shocked, I stared at the film

I chose acupuncture points around his elbows, hips, and back, treating him for Bony Bi in accordance with Chinese medical principles. He grunted and rolled on his side, sleeping during his first acupuncture treatment as the pain was suddenly alleviated. I was somewhat hopeful after witnessing the openness with which he received his first treatment, but then I remembered those nasty radiographs and all that arthritis at such a young age. I did not share my fears with the Sawyers, but I was certain they could read my face. I never was any good at poker.

"What makes this acupuncture stuff work?" Jerry asked. He is a man whose obvious stature and prestige suggest, especially since his graduation into the gray-haired years, that he knows how most things work, like car and ship engines. In fact, I could tell by his pensive glance that when he can't explain how something works, it festers and circles around in his head like a fly trying to find an open window. But the body is not a machine.

I slipped into my acupuncture lecture. "The needles activate nerve pathways that send a signal to the spinal cord and the brain. The specific biochemical workings of that signal are very complex and involve opiate receptors in the spinal cord, and a special interneuron pathway that facilitates communication within the spinal cord itself. Opiate receptors operate in response to acupuncture in a similar manner as they do with drug intervention. It will be some time before we understand the full workings of the nervous system itself, much less every neurochemical reaction that occurs with acupuncture," I said. "For over one hundred years, we did not understand body chemistry enough to explain why aspirin works; we just knew it worked. Now aspirin's prostaglandin inhibitory effect is common knowledge. In fact, many of the pharmaceutical drugs (even prednisone) used today have unknown mechanisms of action. One day, we will be able to explain exactly how acupuncture works."

"Okay, don't tell me about the chemistry, I want to know what acupuncture will do for Denali," Jerry said, growing slightly impatient. The couple wanted results, not explanations.

"This signal tells the spinal cord that the pain it is feeling is not so severe. It also tells the body to stop sending inflammatory chemicals, which cause swelling in the area. The signal tells the spinal cord not to send out so many impulses, and thus muscle spasms are alleviated. The brain receives a message from the needles telling it to release endogenous opiates and enkephalins, which are painkilling chemicals within each of us.

The body has an amazing natural ability to relieve its own pain. Some of these natural endorphins are even forty times more powerful than morphine. They are more powerful than many drugs and, since the body creates them, they are nontoxic."

The Sawyers looked at each other and then at Denali sleeping on the floor and agreed that it must be doing something because "he sure was acting different than normal."

"The needles also make him breathe more deeply, and they make his nose drip." *Now,* I thought, *this will send the Sawyers running!*

Sure enough, Andrea noticed that Denali was breathing more deeply, using his diaphragm, and his nose was dripping away. "Why?"

"His parasympathetic nervous system is being activated." I lowered myself to kneel on the floor. "Those are the things I know about acupuncture, but there is so much about the healing that has no explanation. For example, what makes some animals respond and not others may also have to do with the will of the animal, the intent of the practitioner, and whether or not energy, or Qi, can flow freely. In other words, it will help him if we believe he'll get better."

To my surprise, they were with me on that. After all, they had both prayed at some point, as do most of us if only in fairly desperate situations. I explained that within just a few treatments, we would know whether acupuncture would work for him, but for now, we should remain positive.

"Can't hurt," they both agreed. "I mean, this positive stuff," Jerry added. "But what the heck is Qi?"

"It is life's energy force—that spark when life is first begun. It is what separates the living from the dead. It is the electric, magnetic current that runs in each cell of our bodies," I said. Jerry stared at me and I could see that he needed time to think about our conversation.

We all sat there watching Denali during the twenty-minute acupuncture treatment. Occasionally, one of us would stroke his thick fur. One of the most amazing things about animals is their ability to bridge gaps between very different people. Animals have no ideological boundaries, no political motives, and no judgmental requirements for friendship. For a moment, we forgot our differences. It was very peaceful.

According to Chinese medicine, the dog's red-and-purple tongue, his superficially strong pulses, and his warm creaky joints indicated that he had signs of toxic Heat and Phlegm invading the joints and Stagnating the Sinews. I wanted to cool and detoxify his system but not deplete it, because already the joints were weakened by a lack of vital antioxidant nutrients. Joints receive nutrition and get rid of waste products primarily through movement, and Denali's stiff body indicated that normal cellular metabolic waste products were settling in the joints. This is why arthritis often worsens.

Deposited toxic debris in the body is suspected as one main cause of inflammation because it alters normal tissue chemistry. So I chose to detoxify Denali's body with a largely vegetarian diet: carrots, barley, and just a little white-meat chicken; herbs; vitamin supplementation, especially taurine and vitamin C; kelp; alfalfa; and glucosamine, to help preserve and lubricate the damaged joint cartilage. Dr. Terry Durkes, one of the fathers of gold bead implantation for orthopedic disease, believes that a localized alkalosis in and around joints causes an inability of normal resorption and uptake of calcium as well as destabilizing the vertebrae. Perhaps this is one reason we see diseases such as arthritis and spondylosis in such epidemic proportions, and almost consider them normal in any dog older than five.

Antioxidant vitamins would help repair the free radical and cellular waste product damage affecting Denali's joints as well as exacerbating his seizures. Usually, I recommend only one supplement at a time to avoid the possibility of the patient developing diarrhea, but in Denali's case, we needed to help him fast. With each day, he had been going downhill, and now, together, we had to break that cycle. The Sawyers understood the importance of their involvement and I appreciated this team approach, which is essential for holistic medicine to be successful.

Denali announced that his acupuncture treatment was finished, like most dogs, by standing up, stretching, and shaking his whole body from head to tail, even though he became wobbly. This was a very good sign, because it meant some stagnation was being released. I removed the needles. The Sawyers took Denali home, their minds filled with plans to cook, provide Denali with the supplements, and massage around his joints.

A few days passed and I assumed that despite his positive reaction to the first treatment, the Sawyers had had to put their dog to sleep. Nervously, I called them, and Jerry answered. "Denali?" he said. "Well, he's no worse, so we're sort of happy about that." He added that Andrea was less enthusiastic. Despite the work she put into making his food and giving him his supplements, Andrea still saw Denali falling flat on his nose. She didn't know how long to keep trying, and honestly, neither did I.

At the second treatment, with Denali still holding his left front paw off the ground, the warmth of a rare Seattle sun left us more optimistic. The overgrown shepherd was still unwilling to wag his tail at me, but he was very relaxed with the acupuncture needles, and I was able to needle a few new points on his front feet. I chose points like Triple Heater 3 on the front paws to free the shoulder and elbow from stagnant energy, and Gallbladder 40 on the hind feet to free the stagnant Qi through the shoulders, hips, and knees.

In the third treatment, I combined the acupuncture with chiropractic. After this appointment, Denali went home and slept for hours, as if comatose. In the morning, Jerry poked him to see if he was still alive. Denali didn't stir. But then Andrea yelled at him with her high-pitched Swiss accent, loud enough to wake the dead, and the laid-back dog responded by opening his brown eyes to no more than a squint, barely enough to give her a "leave me alone" look. He got out of his bed, stretched both front and back halves, groaned, and went back to bed.

The Sawyers said that later that day, they could hardly believe their eyes. Not only did Denali walk across the yard, but he ran to play with Jenny, something he had not done for months. In fact, the other German shepherd was so shocked by the surprise attack that she jumped in the air like a cat and bolted forward. Denali was running after her on his front legs, indeed, on all his legs, just like Forrest Gump when his leg braces popped off. Andrea put her coffee down and Jerry wiped his eyes. *It was true—Denali was running!* They called me to report the good news.

"You're kidding, right?" I said, astonished. "How could he be running when he wouldn't even walk three days ago? Is he still falling?" I thought it had to be some kind of joke.

"Well, he's a little funny around corners still, but it's as true as the day is long—that crazy dog is running!" Jerry said, and I heard Andrea calling him in the background. What Denali taught me was that in holistic medical treatment, it's almost impossible to give a prognosis or predict an outcome. The limits I set were only my limits, and often the animal might have more ambitious ideas. It's almost as if some dogs want to get better, and holistic medicine just clears a path for them to heal themselves. All I did was offer a direction for the determined Denali; he himself found the rest of the way.

After the shock wore off, I reflected on the power of acupuncture and wondered if perhaps my tiny acupuncture needles might be electrically connected with a greater universal healing force—the power of which I might never fully realize. So many times I feel that my role in healing is as a facilitator, just a sort of channeler of energy into what I hope is the right direction. I try to maintain a positive outlook, especially since so many of my clients are given negative diagnoses such as "degenerative joint disease" by conventional veterinarians. We can see from Denali's case that "degenerative" does not necessarily mean that the animal will deteriorate.

Four years later, Denali still runs like a puppy. He has not had seizures in all those years. He takes vitamins, glucosamine, and potassium bromide (for the seizures), and, of course, acupuncture/chiropractic treatments every few months. Exercise continues to be a big part of his prescription. Even if dogs are somewhat sore following exercise, keeping the joints moving is very important. This movement helps provide nutrition and removes waste products from the joints as well as strengthening surrounding ligaments and muscles.

Now when I first meet a pet with a severe condition—cancer, heart disease, or advanced arthritis—I think of Denali. I remember how he could not even stand, how he fell rounding every corner, and now how he runs, and runs fast.

Pain

HOW DO I KNOW MY PET IS IN PAIN?

Animals can often exhibit pain very differently from people. Symptoms may include:

- Remaining still, listless, and quiet
- Self-isolation from other animals and people. (Cats commonly hide.)
- Acting needy or more affectionate, or more insecure around other animals
- Crying, howling, or other strange vocalizations
- A worried look in the eyes, showing distress and a sort of bloodshot anxiety.

Genetics determines how easily dogs show pain. Many breeds have been selected to be stoic, or highly pain tolerant. These include many hunting or herding breeds, such as Labradors, pointers, and Border collies. Other breeds—such as huskies and toy poodles—are known to react in an exaggerated fashion to pain if they even anticipate it; these breeds are often known as "pain amplifiers." The best thing to do is stay calm; otherwise, your pet might think things are worse than they actually are.

CONVENTIONAL DIAGNOSTICS

When you take your pet to a veterinarian, let him or her know if your pet's pain is acute or chronic. A physical exam, radiographs, and other diagnostic procedures may expose the cause of the pain. The most common injury I diagnosed on ER was a sprain or other soft-tissue trauma undetectable on films. Blood tests may also be useful in diagnosing chronic pain, because animals with liver or kidney disease or cancer are in pain and might hunch up due to discomfort and weakness, which can easily be misinterpreted as back pain.

What If These Tests Find Nothing Wrong?

You know your pet best, so please persevere. If you think he is in pain, he probably is, even if the veterinarian can find nothing wrong. Western diagnostic tests are valuable once pathologic changes have progressed. Why wait for disease to manifest itself? Holistic modalities help preserve optimum health and can prevent major pathology. Chiropractic exams, acupuncture, herbal therapies, massage, homeopathy, and Bowen therapy (an Australian technique of strumming the muscles to realign the spine) help millions of people—why not give them a try for animals?

HOLISTIC RECOMMENDATIONS

For acute trauma such as bruises and abrasions, try homeopathic *Arnica montana* 30C (see page 259) on the way to the veterinarian. It is readily available at many health food stores and drugstores. Give 3 to 5 pellets as often as every 2 hours until symptoms subside. For chronic back pain that gets worse with exercise, use *Bryonia* 6C; if it gets better with exercise, use

Rhus tox 6C. Try T-touch massage (see Resources, page 266) or massage the affected area yourself, if your pet likes it, in large, soft, slow clockwise circles, making one circle per breath.

Safe Herbal Tea

This is my favorite herbal tea to release muscle spasms, reduce musculoskeletal inflammation, and relieve pain.

 4 cups water or low-sodium chicken broth
 ¼ cup crampbark (*Viburnum opulis*)
 ¼ cup corydalis root (*Corydalis formosa*)
 ¼ cup meadowsweet leaves (*Filipendula ulmaria*)
 ⅛ cup boneset (*Eupatorium perfoliatum*)

Combine all of the ingredients in a small stainless steel or ceramic saucepan, cover, and simmer over low heat for 30 minutes, trying to keep evaporation to a minimum. Turn off the heat and leave the pan covered for 4 to 6 hours. Strain the tea, and discard the solids.

Keeping: The tea will last for up to 2 weeks in the refrigerator. I recommend freezing half of the tea in an ice cube tray, and thawing as needed for later use. Bring to room temperature before using.

Dosing: Give cats 3 cc or about ½ teaspoon twice a day and dogs 1 teaspoon per 20 pounds of body weight either in food or orally, with a syringe. Give until symptoms subside. This does not interfere with other medications, although other medications may be reduced as the pain dissipates.

THE LAST CHANCE DOG

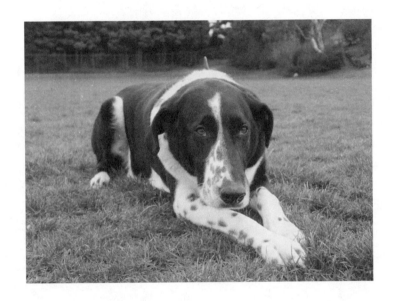

Kincade sports a studded leather collar, weighs 120 pounds, and stands about three and a half feet tall. He's not the type of dog you'd like to annoy. He is black and white, like an Oreo cookie, but the white bits are spotted, as if he is part dalmatian. Nobody knows his breed, but Kade is as unforgettable as his nickname. At least that's what the people say who care for him in the pink rock 'n' roll house where he lives. The house is in one of Seattle's groovy Northside neighborhoods. Molly Clark owns and loves Kade; they also live with Molly's brother, Brent, who's the bass player for the Lemons, and Nicole, a kindhearted blonde who keeps up with the latest hair fashions. Aside from Kade's occasional howls at sirens, it's a pretty quiet part of town—except on the nights when the giant dog seizes. At three years of age, Kade is one of the most violent epileptics I've ever met.

When Kade was a puppy, he got into everything and loved everyone. He tackled bike riders and Rollerbladers with kisses and loved the sound of skateboards, which is good because Brent rode his everywhere. He practiced howling and barking loudly—some say to compete with the electric guitars, but Molly just thinks Kade has a lot to say and wants to be sure people are listening. Like Linus with his blanket, Kade carries the surprisingly tolerant family cat in his mouth. Kade marches up the stairs with the cat's scruff in his teeth to sleep with her on his bed. For some unknown reason, cats follow him wherever he goes.

Other animals like Kade too. Ratty, the family pet white rat, often comes out and crawls all over Kade, who doesn't seem to mind. Brent acquired Ratty when the little fellow clambered over Brent's foot while he was out on the sidewalk. Ratty had had a big gouge in his back and looked as if he had missed a few meals, so the family took him in. Ratty likes to wrap his tail around Molly's neck while balancing on her shoulders.

Molly and her brother are from Chicago. You can tell they are city people by their scratchy voices, their black leather, and their tolerance for noise and chaos. They are both lean and tall. Molly's hair is a variable color, sort of a pink/red brown, short and curly, and it jets in a million directions. And Molly loves Kade more than anyone could imagine. Very few people would have stood by him night after night when he seized, sometimes twenty times in a row. I think her fearless tenacity helps a lot.

Kade usually sleeps at the foot of Molly's bed on his favorite crocheted blanket, and that's where he was the night of "the big one." The neighborhood still gossips about the night of Kade's first seizure. At band practices, the musicians still refer to that night as you would a tornado or a hurricane. Molly knows the date of the big one because it was on Jon Bon Jovi's birthday, March 2, 1997. She had come home from a rock show and cradled Kade's head in her lap for a long time before the two fell asleep.

In the middle of the night Kade suddenly jumped up straight, went stiff, and started bucking like a bronco, pooping and peeing everywhere. Alarmed but still half asleep, Molly nervously touched him, saying, "Are you okay?" But the big dog was as far from okay as he could be.

Kade lunged for Molly, baring his teeth as if possessed by the devil. Molly screamed for help, and Frank, a friend who had crashed that night on their sofa, heard her and ran in. He jumped on Kade's back, trying to wrestle him down. Kade bit his hand, and blood splattered everywhere. Molly threw a stapler at the dog, who went for her again, growling and pinning her in a corner of the room. Molly was trapped and panic-stricken. Her brother and roommates, who were downstairs, screamed up at the possessed dog. Kade clambered down the stairs after them, freeing Molly. He stopped halfway down and ran back up to attack Molly's door, which she had closed. He clawed and bit the door, but thankfully Molly was safe behind it, frozen with fear. Everyone hid behind closet doors or curtains.

Downstairs, Brent armed himself with a frying pan in one hand and a butcher knife in the other, calling Kade nicely and trying to calm him down. Meanwhile, Molly phoned the police, who said they were going to send a sharpshooter to kill the dog. "Hell no!" Molly yelled, and hung up. After a seemingly endless hour with everyone crouched and hiding, Kade returned to his happy, normal self. The roommates crept back out to find Kade looking innocently up at everyone—Frank's bloody hand, Brent with the frying pan, and Molly sobbing—as if to say, "What happened here?"

The exhausted household went on a trip to the emergency room, where the vet took a blood test and then sent the seemingly normal dog home. Afterward, at about four in the morning, they all sat on the tattered beige couch. Molly was committed to saving her dog. "Who's in? Who will support me?" she asked.

"Hell yeah, I love Kade. Well, when he *is* Kade," Nicole said. "Anything for you, Molly." But she eyed the dog suspiciously. Frank said no, he couldn't, and was kicked out of the household pact, but later he changed his mind. By phone, Molly's dad weighed in to say he wanted the dog dead; though he loved Kade, he could recognize that the dog was dangerous. And Kade rested on the floor by their feet like a baby, sleeping. At the moment, the giant dog had never seemed more harmless.

After the first night, the nighttime seizures continued, but they were no longer dangerous to anyone except Kade himself. The giant dog thrust his feet through walls, thrashed his head about, and knocked over furniture. After the seizures, he was blind and moaned for up to two hours. Soon, Molly learned what she had to do—she moved all the furniture out of the first floor, except the soft couch. To keep him from hurting himself, Molly would walk with him for hours, doing laps around the would-be dining room. This seemed to calm him down.

But the seizures continued, and evidence of their impact remains even after several years—urine stains on the red carpet and holes in the walls where Kade's paws pushed through. Only the wall decorations remained, including old posters with legends such as "Zeke, the Lemons, and Slug at the Crocodile." The posters and the lived-in feel of the home gave it the atmosphere of a rock concert mosh pit, but Molly refused to let the band practice there anymore.

Kade's seizures were getting worse. His phenobarbital had been increased to a toxic level: nine pills twice a day. The conventional vet had also prescribed potassium bromide, another anticonvulsant medication, but that made Kade vomit constantly.

Out of desperation, Molly and her dad drove five hours to the College of Veterinary Medicine in Pullman, Washington, where an MRI and a spinal tap revealed no other causes for the violent seizures. "Good news," said the white-coated neurologist who emerged from a back room. "No brain tumor." This was Dr. Rod Bagley, who had been my senior adviser while I was still a vet student and had helped me with the senior presentation that won that year's award, entitled "The Scientific Basis for Acupuncture."

Several years later, Dr. Bagley was a student of mine at the IVAS (International Veterinary Acupuncture Society) veterinary acupuncture course that I helped teach. His scientific mind opened to the world of Eastern medicine, and before you knew it, he was using words such as "Qi" and suggesting diagnoses such as "Liver Fire and Internal Wind."

Back in Pullman, after Kade's MRI, Dr. Bagley explained the Western diagnosis of epilepsy to Molly and her dad, who had waited all day for the results. Idiopathic epilepsy is a "diagnosis of exclusion" and I like to think it's called "idiopathic" because we are idiots and don't know why seizures occur. Although epilepsy affects at least 1 percent of all dogs, the exact neurochemical imbalance that causes it is not known.

This hardly seemed like good news to Molly. To her, the news meant that they were already doing everything they could. Molly had gone months without sleep. Even as Kade rested his large body against her under the covers, she imagined that every twitch was another fit, that every normal dog wiggle was a warning. Those nights she lay frozen, eyes wide open. She could feel the pain of her stomach clenching like an ulcer inside her.

What she imagined was often all too real. She got good at the drill. Feet kicking, teeth chomping, eyes spinning, pooping, peeing, Kade bucked and foamed like a rabid beast. Molly would try to stay straddled on top of him during the bronco episodes so she could catch his head before it hit the floor. The next day, she always went to her veterinarian, who was a wonderfully open and compassionate person but could offer her only one alternative—putting Kade to sleep. If Molly weren't so hardheaded, that's probably what would have happened.

Any change in Kade's environment or diet might have brought on even more seizures. One time Kade got into the garbage and had twelve seizures before Molly gave up and took him to the emergency clinic again. In addition to his regular medication, she also gave him two doses of Valium rectally (no fun task). He stayed at the emergency clinic for the weekend. It cost her two thousand dollars, but they assured her that he would be fine.

That night after he came home, Kade had another seizure in the kitchen. He flipped backward, hit his head on the oven, and fell still, knocked out, blood pouring out of his mouth. His eyes were open, fixed, and he wasn't breathing. Molly called the vet's office and they told her how to do mouth-to-mouth resuscitation. After a few seconds, Kade jolted into a seizure. Blood was spraying and Molly was screaming, until she remembered that no one was home. Another trip to the vet . . .

After racking up seven thousand dollars in veterinary bills on her credit cards, Molly brought Kade to me. I met the whole crew in March 1999: Molly's dad, Brent, Molly, and the mighty and infamous Kade, who trembled in the corner because he was so leery of vets by now. At this point, Kade was seizing one or two times a week. I have never had clients so open to my suggestions. I said, "It is very important that we cut the toxins out of Kade's life. No smoking around him. All-natural, homemade diet, herbs, and a strict exercise program. He should not be around loud music if possible." Molly glanced at her brother. Kade's seizures would turn the rock 'n' roll house into a easy-listening one. We did the first acupuncture treatment, and with needles forming a crown on Kade's head, he stopped shaking and stretched the whole length of the exam room floor to fall asleep.

In Chinese medicine, the three most common causes of epilepsy are Phlegm accumulation, or the buildup of toxins, due, in part, to drugs and vaccines; Blood Stagnation, resulting from head trauma that may even be associated with being born; and Liver Wind, from diet and constitutional predisposition. These patterns can be differentiated by subtle variations in the qualities of the tongue and the pulse, as well as other clinical findings. Many dogs with Liver Wind and seizures also have problems with skin allergies because Wind may also cause itching. It is fascinating that even thousands of years ago, the Chinese knew that when the Liver was in trouble, the body would produce Fire and Wind, which could cause seizures. Now we know this phenomenon as hepatic encephalopathy, and we can measure elevating liver enzymes in the blood.

In contrast to Western medicine, which waits until there are recognizable abnormalities in blood tests or radiographs, Chinese medicine focuses more on the prevention of organ dysfunction by treating small imbalances. Kade's liver enzymes had always been normal, but, unfortunately, by the time blood shows an abnormality, there is already a 70-percent organ dysfunction in all species. Using the subtle principles of Chinese medicine, I checked the abnormalities of his pulse and tongue and diagnosed Liver Fire and Wind.

According to traditional Chinese medical thought, "One should not start digging a well when already thirsty" or "start making weapons when a war has already begun." With this preventive philosophy in mind, I chose points to support the Liver, for its Wind and Fire, and for the Gallbladder, a meridian running through the head. The Gallbladder and the Liver were partners in crime and needed to be balanced. Every dietary and herbal recommendation was aimed at balancing the Liver.

With weekly acupuncture, Kade improved a little—his seizures were less intense and less frequent. We weaned him onto a lower dose of medication. We found that if we waited over a week between acupuncture treatments, he would seize, so Molly decided on gold bead implantation. During this procedure, I thread three to five tiny gold beads into each acupuncture point. It's like permanent acupuncture.

For the procedure, the conventional vet Dr. Windom and I lifted Kade's giant body up onto the steel surgical table. We anesthetized the dog, shaved his head, clipped his hair, and scrubbed the skin clean, just as for any other surgery. I implanted more than a hundred tiny beads at different specific sites on Kade's head, especially on the Gallbladder meridian that crosses the temples. The beads stay under the skin in acupuncture points for the remainder of the dog's life and permanently stimulate the points, so Chinese needles become less necessary. Gold bead implantation is used most commonly for epilepsy, hip dysplasia, and certain spinal conditions.

Kade wore a kerchief around his head for a while, until his hair grew back. Molly could feel the beads under the skin all around Kade's head, and she moved them slightly to stimulate them every day. For a week after the gold beads were implanted, Kade acted sleepy. He seized a few times as he adapted. We did acupuncture once a week again and sat on pins and needles, not knowing the future. At night I thought about poor Kade, who still seemed far from healthy, and questioned myself. I learned that Dr. Terry Durkes had a new technique for implanting gold beads by using pulse diagnosis, and dogs that have cluster seizures, or one right after another, present a more serious problem. According to Dr. Durkes, these dogs may need several more points implanted along the spine. I wondered if Kade needed that or some other variation to improve.

But over the next weeks, the seizures decreased in severity, duration, and frequency, and we saw Kade come back into his own personality. Now that he was no longer on edge because at any moment he could lose control of his body, he rested all night—and so did Molly. After he went two months without a seizure, Molly moved the furniture back into the dining room. Molly and I started referring to the seizures as the "S-word," whispering it so as not to jinx the situation. We held our breath as we slowly weaned him off his medication. Six months later, he went off his herbs, and eventually he stopped coming for acupuncture altogether. The only vestige of Kade's treatment was his homemade diet.

It has been two and a half years since Kade's last seizure. His coat shines due to the homemade food and vitamins. He is not on herbs anymore. Kade plays with the cats again, and sometimes when he hears a siren, he howls with the strength of ten dogs, just so the neighbors have something to talk about.

✺

Seizures

An estimated 1 percent of dogs have epileptic seizures, although this number seems to be growing. Fortunately, cats, horses, and other animals develop the disease less frequently. It is one of the most difficult diseases for human caretakers, because seizures often come on suddenly and violently. Many people have lost sleep worrying about whether their dog would seize. As the Qi circulates its circadian flow of energy through each meridian, it has trouble at night when it reaches the Gallbladder and Liver, normally between eleven P.M. and three A.M.

THE CONVENTIONAL APPROACH
TO SEIZURE DIAGNOSIS

If your pet seizes for the first time, you should immediately see your regular veterinarian. There are two conventional categories for seizures: extracranial, or out of the brain, causes, and intracranial, or in the brain, causes.

Extracranial causes: Blood tests should be done if your pet has never seized before. Low blood sugar caused by infection or insuloma, electrolyte imbalances, or liver abnormalities can cause seizures. These metabolic causes for seizures are very common in cats, who seem to manifest symptoms neurologically.

Intracranial causes: If the blood tests were normal after your pet's first seizure, chances are there is an intracranial cause, namely either a space-occupying lesion (a brain tumor or blood clot), hyperthermia, or brain-swelling disorder, or, finally, epilepsy. If your pet has been diagnosed with epilepsy, holistic care by itself or in combination with conventional drugs may be warranted.

THE DANGERS OF STATUS EPILEPTICUS

During status, animals go into a full tonic/clonic (or twitching), unconscious seizure for a long period of time and may need conventional medication and/or hospitalization. Some dogs do not recover and may suffer brain swelling or other problems from increased body temperature. Lower your pet's temperature with a cool, moistened cloth on the forehead. **Do not put anything in your pet's mouth, especially not your hand!** Administer 4 drops of Rescue Remedy (a Bach flower remedy commonly available at health food stores) plus 5 pellets of *Aconitum* 30C and *Cocculus* 30C (homeopathic remedies) from above the pet's mouth to touch his gums or tongue. If you are using a glass dropper, do not place it in a seizing animal's mouth. Instead drip the contents from above the gums. Go to the veterinarian.

WHEN YOUR PET NEEDS CONVENTIONAL DRUGS

- If his or her seizures are very severe and frequent (more often than one seizure every two weeks).
- If the seizures affect his or her overall personality.
- If the drugs seem to work well, with few side effects. This varies, depending on the animal.

The most common conventional medications to control seizures in animals are phenobarbital or potassium bromide. Some dogs do very well on phenobarbital for many years with little or no apparent liver damage. Sometimes animals must have these drugs to control their epilepsy, but holistic care is an option and can be used in conjunction with these medications.

HOLISTIC METHODS
FOR CONTROLLING EPILEPTIC SEIZURES

These can help control or prevent side effects from medication, keep the dose of conventional drugs lower, and better control seizures.

The following methods can be beneficial:

- a natural diet, especially one supplemented with magnesium (100 milligrams per 40 pounds, unless your veterinarian advises against it—e.g., in cases of renal disease), vitamin E (100 IU per 40 pounds), melatonin (1–2 milligrams before bed if the seizure typically occurs during sleep), and taurine (250 milligrams per 40 pounds)
- maintaining a daily routine, avoiding stress and loud noises
- regular exercise
- herbs, especially the Liver Wind formula Tian Ma Gou Teng Yin; acupuncture; and chiropractic
- gold bead implantation
- logging episodes in a calendar (including time, possible triggers—different food or activity—duration, and intensity) gives your veterinarian valuable information

A helpful website is www.canine-epilepsy.com.

THAT OPEN PLACE

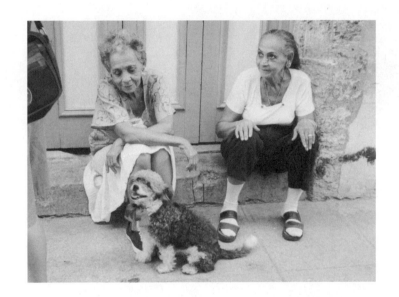

It was a dreary Thursday in November, coming up on another anniversary of my grandmother's death. I was dreading spending another holiday season without her. But animals were still sick, and there was much work to do. A black Lab named Molly was my next patient, and I went out into the clinic parking lot to find her.

"She's been real stiff lately," Michael said, lifting his aged best friend from the trunk of his Subaru. "Maybe it's the weather." He placed her on the concrete and then balanced her carefully on all fours. Arthritis often gets worse in the cold, damp Seattle winters. Gently he placed a towel under her belly and step by step lifted her back legs up to help her walk. She walked as slowly and gingerly as an elderly woman. From her worried frown and pensive gaze, it was clear to me that Molly was upset because her body was deteriorating. She did not whine or whimper, but her tail was lowered; only the very tip of it wagged when she felt obliged to please. Molly tried not to be a bother, but her uncharacteristic silence was the most troubling symptom we faced.

Her hip arthritis was progressing; she now balanced most of her weight on her two front shoulders, pulling her back legs along as if they were a ball and chain. After a treacherous journey up the walkway, which must have seemed like miles, she made it in and sat in front of me, sighing after working so hard. Michael sat on the floor by her side. "Well, the truth is," he said, leveling with me, combing his fingers through his long hair, "I guess she's just not getting any better."

Hearing those words was a veterinarian's worst fear, and they echoed in the exam room as if it were a deep canyon. Over the years, I have seen countless dogs like Molly respond well to acupuncture and herbs, but in front of me sat the reminder of my failed attempts at healing. Her soft and worried stare would haunt me for weeks to come. Some animals are ready to give up—they do not really want to improve, and I believe they are seeking entrance into another spiritual realm. But lately I had treated more patients like Molly, dogs who wanted to improve with all their heart but couldn't. I began to doubt my capabilities. I was frustrated and helpless because I could not find the cause—I blamed myself.

Normally I was optimistic about healing. If chiropractic wouldn't work, I would try acupuncture. If acupuncture wouldn't work, I would try Adequan injections, MSM, glucosamine, herbs, or gold bead implants— all holistic, safe treatments that normally heal animals. But with Molly I found myself saying, "Well, she's old, and her arthritis is so severe . . ." As if I could find solace in making excuses.

Michael nodded and tears welled in his eyes. "If she stops walking, I'll have to put her down. I wish she had cancer or something else— something that seems more serious." Molly nudged his hand over her head. Normally I might have bent down to console Michael and give some words of encouragement. I said nothing. I was numb. It was as if my open, clear conscience had been permeated by a combined sense of loss for my grandmother, and for Molly, and a feeling of hopelessness about my increasingly geriatric practice.

I heard a horrible inner voice say, *How much could poor Molly really improve?* I was starting to sound increasingly pessimistic and had given up on the patients, like Molly, that needed me most. It was as if I had once been part of a powerful cohesive healing force and now, for some reason, had been left to fend for myself—or rather a depressed version of myself.

"Let's treat her today and see how she does," I said, searching my mind for treatment options. The truth was, I was worried that it was no use. I treated her sore hips with acupuncture. After many years of needling patients, I will usually feel a vibration, a warmth or a tingling at my fingertips when the needle reaches the Qi. It is akin to the electrical current of our bodies flowing through the steel acupuncture needle, which acts as a conductor. Without this patient-practitioner energy transfer, healing was less likely to occur. I knew this but couldn't control it. Indeed, it was the last time I ever saw Molly.

Several days later, I dreamed that my house flooded, and as the water rose, my dogs and I struggled to stay afloat. There was a big wall in my backyard and I knew I had to climb over it carrying one dog at a time to save them. I got Sugar, my shepherd cross, over and she collapsed to the ground with fatigue. I went back for Smudge, my smallest older terrier cross. The water was rising faster and the wall was growing too. She still paddled unconsciously in my arms. I could not get over the wall. Every time I got a foothold, the wall grew. I woke still hearing the gush of swirling water and Smudge's labored breathing, which thankfully turned out to be just snoring. I felt powerless and alone. Where could I turn? After all, I was supposed to be the healer.

When Dr. Naomi Bierman, another veterinary acupuncturist from Seattle, called to ask me if I would help teach a twenty-day veterinary acupuncture course in Cuba, a *no* was on the tip of my tongue. I had just settled on the couch in my tiny Seattle house with a dog on each side. I felt stingy with my precious free time. I had just taught in San Diego's IVAS course the year before and was plain tired of traveling. "Why the heck did you choose Cuba?" I asked.

"I can't describe why, but the Cubans are exceptional people. They have a better literacy rate than we do in America. With few resources, they can accomplish great things. It will be the first time an IVAS-endorsed course is offered in a developing country." Naomi added, "Some vets down there have been doing a little acupuncture and a lot of homeopathy for over twenty years already. Maybe we could learn from them." Her voice was focused and unwavering. Naomi is a kind but determined, hardheaded New Yorker—several years of living in Seattle had not drowned her fiery personality.

In the early 1990s, when the Soviet Union collapsed, Cuba entered a "special period" of economic hardship perpetuated by the United States embargo, which essentially excluded Cuba from the world market. Along with medical supplies, farming chemicals also were unavailable. Instead of using pesticides and fertilizers, the Cubans were forced into organic farming and sustainable agriculture. Through imposition came genius—they developed organic farming techniques using draft animals and manure instead of industrial plows and chemical fertilizers.

The Cuban Ministry of Health issued a directive to health care professionals to integrate *medicina verde*—green medicine—into their practices as much as possible. This way the Cubans could grow their own herbs and prepare homeopathic medicine.

Some Cuban doctors use acupuncture, but never had a systemized course in Chinese medicine been taught to the veterinarians there. Since limited finances restrict Cubans from traveling, academic interchange is difficult. To learn veterinary acupuncture in an organized course, the

Cuban veterinarians needed it brought to them. Naomi knew this would be a monumental task, and she needed help.

I paused, still wondering, "Why Cuba?" I told Naomi about my flood nightmare and about my "stuck" feeling, not being fully present with my patients or myself. She suggested that maybe a trip was just what I needed.

"We can't pay anything. The Cubans are rich people but have little money," she said. Naomi had traveled to Cuba six times already to arrange the hotel, students, facilities, and all the massive logistical details that go into arranging a course in a developing country. In Cuba, it is difficult to find pens or paper, much less slide projectors and overhead projectors, so all the equipment had to be brought down. Naomi and Dr. Eric Hartmann, her faithful organizer, had spent months preparing lectures, tinkering with details, and planning the course without receiving any financial assistance.

I looked down at my little dog Smudge. How could I be away from her and Sugar for such a long time? "Naomi, I'll think about it. Cuba sounds interesting, but I am so tired." I hung up the phone and Smudge brought me her favorite toy, a slobber-covered blue octopus that was losing its white cotton stuffing. It was as if she were telling me, "Oh, Mom, quit worrying about me."

Like an estimated 15 percent of all dogs in America, Smudge has skin allergies. Lately, even my acupuncture treatments did not seem as effective. Over the years, she had been doing great with homemade food, herbs, and acupuncture, but recently she itched like crazy. I found bloody lesions on her belly and feet. I felt my ability even to heal my own beloved dog slipping from my grasp.

Being a teaching assistant in Cuba did not sound easy, but I felt Naomi was right—perhaps I needed a change. I told her I would go and help. She smiled when I asked, "But, Naomi, isn't it illegal to go to Cuba?"

"It's not illegal to go, it's just illegal to spend money there," she laughed. "But don't worry, we are going legally, under guidelines established by the U.S. Treasury Department for professional exchanges.

"Donna, you aren't going to believe this. Every holistic veterinarian I asked to teach in Cuba agreed to help—without financial assistance of any type. And I asked sixteen of you," Naomi said. It was amazing that so many would help knowing they would have to cover all expenses plus lose revenue while away from their practices. I still had mixed feelings. I remember thinking: *Okay, so a bunch of us are crazy.*

A few months later, I found myself packing for the trip. I received a list of odd necessities. Packages of Kleenex, bottles of ibuprofen (which I almost never take), feminine hygiene supplies, sixty boxes of acupuncture needles, packages of pens, huge ten-packs of soap, paper . . . Thankfully, at the last minute I threw in some soy protein powder and rice milk. I am a strict vegetarian, and I was told vegetarian food might be scarce. Actually, Eric Hartmann told me, "Donna, you're gonna starve." I assumed he was exaggerating. I filled my suitcases thinking that I wouldn't use any of the supplies myself but that I could leave what we did not use with the Cubans. I wondered how I would hand a Cuban vet a package of Kleenex. How could these cheap gifts be useful to anyone?

All the empty corners of my bags I filled with pharmaceutical drugs. I combed my house to find what we holistic vets love to call the "antis," or drugs that work against the natural tendencies of the body. I packed amoxicillin (an antibiotic), phenylbutazone (an anti-inflammatory), Pepto-Bismol (an anti-spasmodic), and ivermectin (an anti-parasitic). Some holistic vets were even calling drug distributors in a desperate attempt to acquire as many drugs as possible. How ironic that proponents of natural medicine were scrounging for conventional medical donations! The experience made me realize that although I use conventional drugs at home only as a last resort, they're sure good to have sometimes. In America, I had grown weary of the excessive use of pharmaceutical drugs, but in Cuba these drugs were essentially unavailable and sorely needed. Every bottle I packed might save a life, help a family, or stop the painful constant itch of canine mange.

Dr. Christine Susumi, another veterinarian and acupuncture teacher, and I traveled together, and since direct flights from the United States to Cuba are very hard to come by, we went through Cancún. We had to leave plenty of time to get through customs with the massive amount of medical donations Chris had brought.

On the plane trip, I wondered what Cuba would be like. I wondered and I worried. My Spanish skills were pretty shabby. What if this healing crisis affected my teaching too? If there was a subject I could worry about, I managed to let my thoughts dwell there on that plane ride. But somewhere between the snack service on the Cancún-bound flight and my discovery of colorful piñatalike figurines at the Mexican airport stores, I stopped worrying.

At three in the morning, Chris and I finally arrived in our room in

Havana at the Hotel Ambos Mundos—Both Worlds Hotel. The bellhop whispered directions in muffled, broken English on how to use the room safe. We were trying not to wake anyone. All at once the safe slipped from its weakened hold on the wall and slammed to the floor, its impact echoing through the hushed hotel like an explosion. The bellhop, Chris, and I laughed heartily at the momentary awkwardness. I knew Cuba would be interesting, if nothing else. That was the first time I had laughed in quite a while.

At first, all I saw in Havana was the poverty. The streets were humid and hot and busy with all sorts of people, many of whom were thin and begged for money. Food was limited, by most standards. The dilapidated buildings were intriguing because their infrastructure was crumbling away around the solid marble, stone floors, and archways that had once been so grand. The embargo and the resulting poverty wreaked havoc with the beautiful architecture. There was limited paint and other construction supplies.

But after a few days, I saw beyond Havana's rough surface to something more powerful about the city and its people. Gradually, the open, natural warmth and vibrant energy of the people began to rub off on me. I saw past the poverty. I saw old men singing to themselves and swiveling to their private tunes. Women with skintight, colorful striped Lycra pants danced, free from self-consciousness.

I found Havana to be a rich, seductive center of human vitality, full of spirits, some living, some dead, some content, others restless. I wandered the streets of old Havana, staring up at the buildings. Havana, under Castro, is extremely safe by American standards, so even at night, I did not mind being alone. I could speak to people and improve my awful Spanish. Knowing little about architecture, I nonetheless appreciated the beautiful stone columns, ornate carved pillars, and iron-laced balconies cluttered with plants and hanging laundry. I especially noticed the smell of diesel fuel that keeps the old 1950s American cars running. The age of many of the cars marks the beginning of the U.S. embargo, more than forty years ago.

In Cuba, I reflected on how different life was in the States, where we work on ways to be alone—to live individually, to make decisions with primarily our own well-being in mind. We go to therapists, end relationships if they don't benefit us, and move to different states to achieve career goals. We might even medicate ourselves in order to cope with the pressures of operating individually, our loneliness accruing. But in Cuba, people freely admit that they are nothing without each other. They touch each other, they hug perfect strangers, and they see the beauty in just being with other people. I realized that at home I was not part of a community of healers, and that I had lost track of my mentors.

In Cuba, I met one of them again. Dr. Cheryl Schwartz didn't know it, but she was the reason I had become an acupuncturist in the first place. I can remember one afternoon while I was still a high school student. I had come home from school, just like all the other boring days, broken open a bag of Cheez-Its, and plopped myself in front of the television. (Now I do not eat Cheez-Its and I don't watch television.) There was my future colleague, a vivacious lady with short platinum blond hair and long dangly earrings, treating a poodle with acupuncture. All I remember thinking was how strange the whole thing seemed and that she must have drugged the dog to make him put up with all those needles! But in vet school, when teachers spoke of the side effects of various medications, a distinct vision of Cheryl and the poodle came into my mind. Little did I know, that day, on my couch in Federal Way, Washington, that several years later I would also be threading acupuncture needles into my own dog patients' key points and speaking of their Qi flow.

Now she was in Cuba with me, teaching the Cuban veterinarians as she had once taught me during the early 1990s. In Havana, Cheryl and I and fifteen other veterinary acupuncturists taught veterinarians from many nations including Austria, Canada, Puerto Rico, Poland, Chile, the Netherlands, and Brazil, as well as, of course, the United States and Cuba. We talked about a new way to think about veterinary medicine—according to the principles of traditional Chinese medicine. In the crowded and humid conference area of Hotel Ambos Mundos (famous as one of Ernest Hemingway's residences in Havana), with the help of a Spanish interpreter, we brought veterinary acupuncture to Cuba. It struck me as odd that Chinese medicine was taught in English and then translated into Spanish. Altogether, we were eighty veterinarians from all over the world with one common goal—achieving better animal health through acupuncture.

The cross-cultural differences among the veterinarians were striking. So many things we American vets take for granted our Cuban counterparts greatly appreciated. Since I had recently been bitten in the face by a dog, I decided to bring a few muzzles to Cuba for laboratories because I didn't know how the Cuban dogs would take to having several vets gently touch them. The Cuban veterinarians had apparently never seen a muzzle and immediately began investigating the strange devices. Within a few minutes, a group of four or five Cuban vets were gathered around them and drawing up plans for making their own muzzles from leather! Those plans looked like an architectural drawing, detailed and drawn to proportion.

Another group of Cuban veterinarians said they were planning to make their own acupuncture needles. I was amazed by the dedication and skill with which they figured out ways around obstacles that might have stumped me. Hearing their thanks every day, I felt so appreciated, so much a part of a healing effort that was important on a global scale.

There were as many Cuban women veterinarians as men and the group was racially diverse as well. Many of them were teachers themselves, heads of vet schools, leaders in veterinary associations, chicken vets, cattle and horse vets, and dog and cat vets too. By day we taught; by night we explored the city. Cheryl, Eric, Chris, Naomi, and I danced, in my case a rather stiff gringo version of salsa, to amazingly vibrant African-influenced Latin music. We drank *mojitos,* lime and mint drinks made with white rum. I wasn't sure if it was the music or the warmth and generosity of a people who have so little, but something opened my heart more every day and all my emotions came more easily than they had at home. I felt like myself. If I saw a sweet, bald dog on the street, I would weep. If something struck me as funny, I would laugh openly, without restraint or the sort of self-consciousness I had become accustomed to in the States. There was a sense of acceptance in Cuba without regard to material possessions. It was also easier to live in the present, to appreciate the moment. Soon I left my wristwatch off at night, and lost myself in the music of the streets.

I will always remember how the spirits in Havana took many forms— statues of men and women intertwined, reinforcing and empowering one another. The spirits lived in strange curly-tailed comical lizards that buzzed along like cartoon characters and in stray dogs that walked with purpose. There were spirits that lived in the people's dance and in the old buildings that could tell generations of stories. Havana is a city that can heal, where people come to find something inside them that was lost. Artists come for inspiration; writers find their muse again; musicians can feel new rhythms enter their bones.

One night, I went out to dinner with a small group of American veterinary acupuncture students and a few teachers. Walking arm in arm down Obisbo Street toward the Floridita Hotel, we all felt spiritually connected to one another, as if invisible forces had cast a magic spell over us. It took us all in, charmed us as the Cuban men do, and before I knew it, after a few *mojitos,* we were all swiveling from the waist down. I relaxed muscles I did not even know were tense. I spoke for hours with the other holistic vets about energy pathways, animals we had healed, and those, like Molly, that we could not heal. Together we felt enchanted, and I felt part of a cohesive healing effort and empowered by it.

At one in the morning, a gangly, oily street dog met us at the door of our hotel. He was a brindle hound with toughened skin and a strong constitution. A long but superficial gash bled on the top of his head. All at once, we moved to help him. Using an antibiotic herbal ointment, I treated his wound. While Dr. Jay McDonnell, a neurosurgeon from Tufts University School of Veterinary Medicine, who went to Cuba as an acupuncture student, held his head, I spread anti-parasitic medicine on his back. The medicine would help him with any type of skin parasite—fleas, mites, or lice.

The next night we treated some more street dogs and I did acupuncture on a carriage horse with a swollen fetlock joint above his hoof. I struggled to communicate with the cowboy that I needed him to take all the tack off the horse. Finally, I asked, *"Sin ropas, por favor,"* because my Spanish was so poor. Everyone laughed because my request was, translated, "Naked, please." I blushed and turned to the students, saying, "At least he knew what I meant!"

We treated them not for money, but for that warm feeling that comes when you help animals. I realized when I turned to walk over the cobbled streets that in Havana I was falling in love. Not with a man, but with a new open place within my core. I realized that I was still opening, still evolving, and still had the best asset in being a healer—my beginner's mind. The strength of healing energy must be tended and rekindled by community.

At the end of the acupuncture course, I worked with a Cuban vet, Dr. Jesus Vivanco Puyada. Since he was already an expert in herbal and homeopathic medicine, acupuncture was a natural next step in his small animal practice. He successfully used herbal soaks for chicken with infected feet, and homeopathy for cows with mastitis. After the "special period," Dr. Jesus and his wife, who is also a veterinarian, switched to a dog and cat practice because of popular demand. He earns about twelve dollars a month, which is not much, but the Cuban government supplies the bare necessities—housing, food, education, and health care.

I joined Dr. Jesus at his home, where we treated animal patients on his living room floor. Along with the rest of the family—his wife, two daughters, and his mother—he hugged me as he welcomed me into his house. On small paper plates, they offered me all the food available that day— amazing sweet, large mangos and papayas.

There were no shelves piled high with pharmaceutical supplies, as in the States, and Jesus simply sat on the pink-and-black marble floor of his home in Santa Maria, about fifteen miles outside Havana. Outside, cars sped by a few feet from the front door, while slower horse-drawn carriages also made their way down the street. These carriages are still a primary mode of transportation outside large cities. It was loud with the front door open but much too hot to close it.

Smiling, always smiling, Dr. Jesus tapped his large dark-rimmed glasses closer to the bridge of his nose and rolled up the sleeves on his red-and-white-striped cotton shirt. His body language was warm and open. It was time to get to work. I sat on a chair by his side, and in walked his first patient of the day, Negrita, a seven-year-old furry, dark gray terrier. Negrita's human, Susana, was also a graying middle-aged woman who looked deeply troubled.

Negrita had skin allergies and recurrent ear infections. Parasites are very common in Cuba because of the heat and weakened immune systems caused by poor nutrition—something the tiny bugs thrive on. Immediately, I thought of Smudge and all my dog patients at home that also scratch. For them, parasites are not usually to blame but, instead, stress on the liver from too many drugs, vaccines, and chemicals.

"*Sube aqui*" ("Come up"), Susana said to Negrita, and to my surprise, the small dog did jump up on the chair beside her. Dr. Jesus read the lab report, which described the organisms growing in her ears: "*Conclusiones: De los exudados oticos*—Staphylococcus aureus. *Sensible a: Eritromicina, Tetraciclina, Kanaomicine . . . Resistente a Penicilina . . .*"

I had never seen a lab report or any of the antibiotic names in Spanish! But why did the Cubans bother to make a culture and sensitivity report when antibiotics were not accessible and not affordable? Dr. Jesus blushed when I asked him and shrugged humbly. "We still want to practice medicine," he said. I was touched. What courage it must take to face your job every day knowing helpful medicines exist but are out of reach. But Dr. Jesus wanted no sympathy. His medicines did not come from a drug cabinet—they came from his own backyard.

For traditional herbalists in Cuba, spirituality and medicine are one and the same. Orishas, or Santeria saints, govern the plants and help guide their medicinal abilities within the body. For example, Orisha Osain is the god of all plants, the king of the bush. Being without parents, he sprang up from the soil, according to folklore, and is very conscious of the way he looks. His head is oversized and hidden behind a mask of straw. He is malformed and his ears are asymmetrical, one very big and deaf and the other tiny and so hypersensitive that it can hear a leaf fall on the other side of the world. Many Cuban herbalists sing to Osain when they work with herbs.

I felt sad that Dr. Jesus did not have anti-parasitic drugs, but he could help the dog without them. I followed Dr. Jesus through his long one-story house. There are no doors on any of the bedrooms so I peered into each one. The blankets were old and tattered. The colors were dingy, and the paint was peeling. There were hundreds of flies in the kitchen and no running water that morning. As in most Cuban homes, there was no toilet paper. Rows of chickens in small cages lined an outdoor room. In the backyard, I saw Jesus's medicinal herbs—Mexican sugarcane (used for kidney stones), a guayaba tree (for respiratory disorders), and manzanilla, or chamomile. He was also blessed with a large mango and a large coconut tree, on which the family depended for food.

We cut some guayaba and manzanilla leaves for Negrita's herbal tea and returned to the small shaggy terrier in the front room. To strengthen the dog's immune system and offer her some instant relief from the itching, Dr. Jesus wanted to do an acupuncture treatment. He looked at me. I knew acupuncture was new to him and reassured him that I would help.

In typical Latin fashion, there were no time restrictions for our appointment with Negrita. Jesus smiled; he was so present. There was nowhere he needed to go and no phone to interrupt. His sincere kindness and pure healing intent were as fresh as a fall breeze on a hot Cuban day. The animals responded to him openly as well, knowing he would take the time to empathize with them.

Dr. Jesus spoke with Susana for a long time, softly stroking Negrita's ears without realizing it. Susana began to weep, and then to sob softly. Her son had just moved to Miami, and she did not expect to hear from him for a long time, maybe never. Things were so hard in Cuba; how could she blame him? Now all she had in the world was Negrita, who, perhaps feeling the pressure of promotion to "only household companion," had started scratching almost neurotically. Dr. Jesus spoke quietly to Susana. I didn't understand him, but whatever he said must have comforted the woman because she relaxed deeper into her armchair.

When Dr. Jesus gently flipped Negrita over to scratch her belly, the terrier's back leg started the unconscious twitch of an itchy dog. Working side by side with Dr. Jesus, I felt Negrita's pulses on one back leg and Dr. Jesus felt the other. *"Que piensas?"* ("What do you think?") I asked.

"Deficiencia" ("Deficiency"), he answered. Yes, the small dog's pulses were weak and choppy, indicating a Qi and Blood deficiency, possibly from parasitism or poor nutrition. Her tongue was slightly pale. Dr. Jesus and I looked at each other. *"Los puntos"* ("The points"), he said, and I knew, just as at my practice so many miles away, he was trying to think of all the acupuncture points that would be helpful. We had to nourish her Blood and tonify her body.

"Higado tres" ("Liver 3"), he said, and looked at me. I pointed to the location of Liver 3, on the inside of the back paws. This was a great point for Negrita, because according to the principles of Chinese medicine, if the Liver is not healthy enough, it can't supply ample Blood to the skin. Together we chose other points to extinguish Wind, nourish Blood, and harmonize Liver, all of which should help with the itching.

It was gratifying when Negrita fell asleep, even with the whizzing traffic going by. Susana commented that the needles had a relaxing effect; this was the longest time Negrita had gone without scratching. Dr. Jesus instructed her on how to make the herbal bath, and he prescribed the homeopathic medicine *Chamomila* 30C. He was very experienced with this form of holistic medicine, and I took notes on all his herbal and homeopathic suggestions. We were a good team, he and I; even though my Spanish was limited, as was his English, we communicated with a combination of charades, Spanglish, and good intent. People laughed when they saw us flapping our arms or scratching at ourselves to mimic patients.

Dr. Jesus had a friend who made more money driving a taxi than he did in his medical practice. The two men drove me back to my hotel in a refurbished gold 1950s Chevy with a compact disc as the rearview mirror. They dropped me off on the famous Malecon, the avenue that passes along Havana's ocean side. I kissed Dr. Jesus goodbye. He shed tears as we embraced and I had a lump in my throat as we parted. I promised to bring his wife some grooming books and his daughter some candy when I returned.

I walked back to my hotel on old cobblestone roads, passed Spanish forts, and stepped between the cannonballs that lined the pedestrian-only streets. While I packed to return home, I thought of Dr. Jesus on his floor with Negrita. I felt inspired by his humility and by his integrity. He was a true healer.

When I returned to my clinic, I looked up at my shelves of herbal medicine. Seeing Dr. Jesus in his medicinal garden motivated me to weed my own and spruce it up. I wanted to use more fresh herbs in my practice and rely less on bottled medicines. I was so happy to see Smudge and Sugar. After a few days, I did acupuncture on Smudge for her skin allergies. As I put the small needles into her skin, I thought about Dr. Jesus, Negrita, and the itchy Cuban street dogs.

As if my own healing touch had returned, I felt the energy between my fingers and Smudge's needles vibrate slightly. This sensation, called De Qi, often predicts a great outcome in Chinese medicine. Like dance partners, the patient and the practitioner often feel the energy exchanged. It was as if I had been released from the grip of grief and isolation and allowed to dance again—a sacred healer's dance with Qi's life energy. Without realizing it, Negrita and Dr. Jesus helped me regain my healing touch, and Havana helped restore my open heart.

Coping with Allergies

Allergies have reached almost epidemic proportions in dogs and cats. In conventional terms, the most common allergens are flea saliva, foods, and inhaled airborne particles such as pollen and molds.

Dogs with atopy, or inhaled allergies, are often hard to treat. Commercial diets, hyposensitization injections, antihistamines, shampoos or sprays, and steroids do help some pets but may offer only temporary relief. While corticosteroids seem miraculous in the short term, they often only irritate the immune system over time, driving the body deeper into pathology. Long-term steroid therapy leads to the most serious diseases—Cushing's syndrome, diabetes, and other often hard-to-reverse illnesses. Dogs with skin allergies often develop chronic ear infections and secondary bacterial skin infections, and seem tired because so much of their energy is spent scratching their itches. They can also be irritable and grouchy. Allergies can change a pet's personality. There are thousands of itchy dogs for whom conventional medicine offers no help.

Skin allergies in cats may be present as miliary dermatitis with little bumps and crusty scabs forming on the neck and back. Skin allergies can be one cause of hyperesthesia, a condition in which the nerves of the back appear overstimulated. Cats afflicted with hyperesthesia and intense skin allergies may exhibit symptoms elicited by even the softest touch, including strange skin ripples or seizurelike episodes of frantic racing, panic, or biting at the air.

The way I explain allergies is that the body reacts inappropriately to things it shouldn't react to. The immune system, which has been designed to attack viruses and bacteria, thinks that the antigens (dust, etc.) are like a virus and might attack the body. So it calls in the troops and the pet's skin becomes a front line, where, silently, a war is fought. The red skin and heat are actually your pet's own inflammatory cells—the frontline soldiers who believe they are protecting the pet from invasion when they are really causing the ruckus themselves. Holistic veterinarians tend to focus less on all the potential allergens of the world and more on regulating the immune system.

If conventional medicine has proved to be frustrating, try to consult a holistic veterinarian schooled in acupuncture, herbs, nutrition, and NAET (www.naet.com), Nambudripad's Allergy Elimination Technique, which is a system of diagnosing and treating specific allergens by shifting the body's energetic control of the immune system. It is explained thoroughly in "White Poodle Blues" (page 229).

Holistic medicine can help most animals if the pets' owners are patient enough. Natural alternative treatments often take longer but offer permanent cures.

CATCH THE SYMPTOMS EARLY

The earlier a pet sees a holistic veterinarian, the better. Even though I have seen improvement in pets who have been on daily steroid therapy for years, it often takes a long time to help them holistically. Steroids are very damaging, as they deeply suppress the immune system. Symptoms mount upon the immune system the way an onion grows layers. Natural approaches can be used to peel each layer back in order to find and treat each problem at its core.

Allergies usually develop when the pet is around two or three years of age. Perhaps you notice your cat sneezing for prolonged periods, or your dog scratching his face on the carpet and then chewing on his paws. Horses get allergies too and might rub their heads on stall doors or chew at their flanks. You might notice hives or urticaria, numerous bumps or hot spots on the skin.

If you cannot consult a veterinarian, try antihistamines and diet changes first. In cats, chlorpheniramine (2 milligrams twice a day); in dogs, Benadryl, diphenhydramine (25 milligrams per 50 pounds), or hydroxyzine as prescribed by your veterinarian. These oral antihistamines may help some animals and are very safe to try, the worst side effect being drowsiness. Try natural diets using potatoes instead of grains. According to NAET testing, many dogs and cats have grain allergies, even to rice! Act to help your pet while the symptoms are in their earliest phases, because allergies tend to worsen as your pet ages.

In addition to natural diets, antihistamine therapy, and limiting vaccinations, try using the homeopathic remedy *Urtica urens* 30C (nettles), giving 3 pellets once every 5 days, for a total of three doses. As with all homeopathic remedies, do not touch the pellets, because this can interfere with the treatment. This remedy is available at health food stores or homeopathic suppliers. Give it on an empty stomach.

Try green tea baths and rosemary and chamomile shampoos. Since allergies are so complicated, it is easiest to work with a holistic veterinarian if there is one in your area. NAET, acupuncture, herbs, and constitutional homeopathy have helped thousands of itchy pets when conventional skin testing, hyposensitization, and corticosteroid therapy have failed.

MIKEY'S ON OVERDRIVE

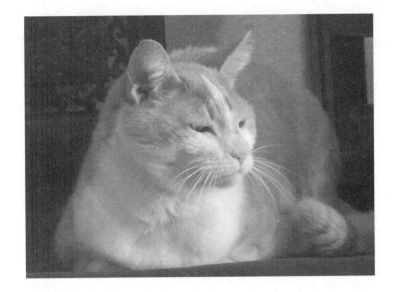

Mikey oversees my waiting room like a feline Dalai Lama, gracing us with his all-knowing presence. Each time I treat the sixteen-year-old tabby, he runs into my waiting room and jumps on his chosen throne—his favorite antique Chinese hand-carved rosewood chair. He doesn't bother sitting on people's laps; after all, he can't really analyze you that way. Instead he meets your gaze from a few feet away, with a wise receptivity that makes you want to leave gifts at his feet and humbly ask him for answers to the world's most pressing questions. Mikey is the only cat I've ever met who actually talks. His meows have the same intonation as sentences. In fact, I feel it is my lack of fluency in cat rather than his weak English that limits our full exchange of language.

Mikey's human father is Trip Quillman, a tall, thin, intellectual psychotherapist with glasses and a sporty, get-things-done-type persona. Trip is the most emotionally perceptive person I know, and his ability to create a safe place for his clients to explore their emotional senses has clearly spilled over to Mikey. Once, while I trimmed the cat's nails, I smiled to hear Trip's voice across the exam table: "Don't hold in your anger, Mikey!" And the orange cat didn't. He yowled at us in discontent and then quickly let it all go, retiring with a deep purr once we were through.

Although Mikey is a calm, interactive cat, a few months before I met him he was quite the opposite—pacing, meowing, and anxious. He had a hyperactive thyroid gland that worked overtime, pumping out an excess of metabolism-increasing hormones. Mikey's symptoms could be attributed to a disorder known as hyperthyroidism, but ultimately it was his emotional and spiritual strength as well as holistic medicine that cured him.

Unlike Mikey, Trip is a natural introvert. Mikey has always been a cat who takes action when he's lonely; Trip wishes he could do the same. Over the years, the neighbors have known more about Mikey than about Trip.

"How's Mikey?" they ask over the fence. "Haven't seen him in the last few days." Trip strives to become more like his cat. He has written notes to himself as if they're from Mikey and posted them on the refrigerator: "Get to know the neighbors"; "Make plenty of friends"; "Find a way out of this loneliness"; "Even if your hips are sore, take a walk every day."

Once Trip told me, "It's like living with a movie star. Mikey is always trying to force me to become more outgoing, to mingle more, and to commit myself." Trip has learned a lot about commitment since he and Mikey have been together. By adopting a cat, after all, he had dedicated himself to Mikey's care for the next twenty years. "It's a daunting responsibility."

Trip first noticed Mikey's medical problems after they lost Lilian, Mikey's sister. For years, the siblings had slept wound around each other. Living in a bachelor's pad with dying houseplants and nothing in the refrigerator except cat food, beer, and a carton of old Chinese takeout was not always so easy. Sometimes the two cats revolted, crying and howling to reprimand Trip when he returned from work late at night. Once Trip had to climb a spruce tree in the backyard to retrieve one of his pouting felines. Although he'd always been healthy, after Lilian died, Mikey became less resistant to illness. Trip recalled Mikey's loneliness—searching the house for hours for his deceased sibling.

The notion that emotional disruption causes physical disease is not new. According to the laws of Chinese medicine, excessive or manic joy can injure the Heart. Excess worry damages the Spleen and can interfere with digestion. Anger, resentment, and frustration are associated with Liver Stagnation or Fire, while fear and shock attack the Kidney, and excess grief can injure the Lung. Unlike the traditional Western medical belief that psychological disease is distinct from bodily pathology, according to the principles of Chinese medicine, the two are interdependent.

All too often, pets absorb the emotional disharmony within a household. When people fight, animals try to break it up or hide from yelling and angry words. Over time, fighting with your family or partner, social isolation, depression, and many other human emotional hardships will harm pets as well.

Being a particularly astute chap, Trip knew that loneliness was affecting Mikey. When Trip would leave for longer than normal periods of time, Mikey's repressed frustration would occasionally cause cystitis, or an inflamed bladder. I knew this symptom well, because many people complain that when they pull suitcases out to pack for a trip, almost instantly, their cats begin to howl painfully in the litter box. The pain is often accompanied by blood in the urine. Although diet can play a role in urinary tract disease, emotional distress is an especially important predisposing factor.

Many holistic veterinarians believe that cystitis develops through the Chinese concept of Liver Qi Stagnation, or anger, which blocks the smooth flow of Qi. This blockage causes energy to slow down and heat up. The accumulation of Heat then sinks down to the bladder, causing a burning sensation. The Heat also makes the Blood "reckless" and drives it out of the vessels and into the urine.

Problems really escalated when a stray cat found its way into Trip and Mikey's house through the cat door. That cat was an unneutered male and peed all over the house that foul, potent, rank-smelling urine particular to tomcats. Imagine the indignity of having your own private territory not only invaded but marked by a total stranger! As Trip spent long hours cleaning up the urine and cursing the stray cat, Mikey began pulling out large clumps of his own hair in protest. Days later, Mikey continued to grab large tufts of his belly hair and angrily pulled it out. Their regular vet prescribed Valium.

Despite medication, the problem persisted and Trip worried about Mikey. Ever since the peeing stray-tomcat invasion, Mikey ate less, yowled at the windows, and displayed all the symptoms that caused Trip to diagnose his human clients with post-traumatic stress disorder. The cat's self-esteem plummeted. To add insult to injury, some squirrels decided to take advantage of Mikey's weakened state and moved into the attic, scratching and pattering about all night long.

Trip commented, "I still feel bad about those squirrels. I just couldn't call an exterminator, so we lived with them for a whole winter. It just tortured poor Mikey."

Mikey had trouble sleeping. Whereas a few months before, the extroverted feline had occupied himself by walking down to the local grocery store to greet customers as they entered, he now isolated himself. He withdrew even from Trip, hiding under the bed or in closets. He was uninterested in his favorite catnip toys or raising a ruckus over the squirrels.

During repeated trips to his veterinarian, Trip discussed Mikey's symptoms. They had decided that Mikey lived in constant fear of another stray-cat invasion, so together the veterinarian and Trip formulated a very unconventional plan. Late at night, when he was sure the neighbors were asleep, Trip went out in the front yard and peed on the bushes to help mark Mikey's territory and scare away cat thugs. It was a last-ditch effort to bolster the protective potency of Mikey's urine.

At times, Mikey seemed to grow a little irritated with Trip's attempts to support his feline psyche; but at least for now, Trip and Mikey were safe from stray-cat confrontations. Perhaps by coincidence, the squirrel family moved out. Slowly, in spite of his embarrassment that his urine had somehow lost its potency, Mikey overcame his anxious behaviors. But Mikey was still physically ill, haunted by recurring vomiting, weight loss, and urinary tract infections. After several weeks of self-conditioning, despite his slipping health, Mikey emerged from hiding places to visit with neighbors and go to the local grocery store again.

The two bachelors grew closer than ever. Each day when Trip returned from work, he saw Mikey waiting on the front steps. The cat would dart down the steps upon seeing Trip back the car in the driveway, and rear up on his hind legs to greet Trip, like a toy poodle. At night, they slept together.

Of all the symptoms, Trip was most concerned about Mikey's weight loss. Although Mikey was increasingly hungry and thirsty, he had lost three pounds within the past two months. He paced, yowled, and had trouble sleeping. His coat dried out, and his spirit faded. More than ever, Mikey sought out wet showers or sinks and would often sit in a shallow puddle of water. He loved olive oil, and he'd often leap onto countertops to drink some. It was as if he was trying to quell a fire within his body.

Mikey was diagnosed with hyperthyroidism, or thyrotoxicosis, by their regular vet, a condition in which the gland's overproduction of the thyroid hormone has toxic effects on the body. The thyroid gland is close to the Adam's apple, in the center of the neck. Excess levels of the thyroid hormone cranked up Mikey's metabolism, making him eat, yowl, drink, vomit, pee too much, and suffer from insomnia. Wandering around at night, Mikey would yowl restlessly. He pulled his hair out in clumps, and he lost so much weight Trip could scarcely recognize his bare, skeletal form. After Mikey's thyroid went into overdrive, all the cat's efforts went into bodily functions instead of the spiritual attunement for which he had become famous.

Feline hyperthyroidism is a maddening disease. It is extremely common, currently the number-one endocrine disease in middle-aged cats. Although Western and Eastern doctors have different strategies for treating this disease, we do agree that the heart and kidneys are affected and that the fluids of the body dry up, becoming consumed by heat. What causes the disease? Why is it so common in cats and not in dogs? Conventional medicine is still searching for a cause, sometimes referring to the overactive thyroid gland as a tumor. Typically, mainstream vets do not mean a cancerous tumor that can spread, but rather that the cells of the thyroid gland overreplicate and overproduce thyroxin. The gland enlarges because it is overactive.

According to Chinese medicine, the disease is preceded by several events. Many holistic vets believe commercial cat food is to blame, especially the fat used to coat the kibble in order to improve its taste. Many months to years before cats are diagnosed with hyperthyroidism, possibly from eating overly oily commercial cat food, they often show signs of accumulation of Dampness because of the Spleen's inability to completely transform the food into Qi and usable body fluids. The body is unable to use Dampness as it does normal fluids. Common symptoms include vomiting, diarrhea, and hair loss on the belly from constant licking or grooming. The tongue is swollen and wet with strings of saliva. Cats are supposed to eat mice, or at the very least a home-prepared diet, not dry kibble cat food. Switching from dry or canned commercial food to homemade food is much more difficult to do with cats than dogs. Cats are addicted to the taste of the fat added by commercial pet-food manufacturers and often refuse a homemade diet. My clients with the most success literally trade one kibble at a time for equal amounts of home-cooked food, so the conversion takes about a month.

Dry kibble can whisk water away from the body, drying out the body's Yin, or fluids, and weakening the Kidneys over time. A deficiency of Yin impairs the body's ability to cool, moisten, and nourish. The balance between Yin and Yang is disrupted; Yang becomes excessive, and the body heats up. In Western medicine, the parasympathetic nervous system is Yin, responsible for digestion, rest, and bodily excretions, while the sympathetic nervous system is more Yang. It includes the flight-or-fight aspect of the nervous system.

Dampness and Yin deficiency make the body heat up. This excess Heat enters the Blood and is circulated to all parts of the body, eventually becoming trapped in different locations. Core body temperatures may increase. This may be one cause of the conventional diagnosis of "fever of unknown origin," which is common in cats. The Liver struggles to detoxify and cool the Blood, but cannot keep up, elevating liver enzymes on blood tests. Cats may be more afflicted with hyperthyroidism because they tend to heat up and dry out more easily than dogs. Sometimes clients say their cat feels hot to the touch.

Even if the body temperature remains normal, at this point in early Yin deficiency, owners may not notice much—the cat might drink a little extra water. There is no weight loss, and the coat may be dry, which is not unusual for cats. Then, suddenly, seemingly overnight, cats begin to drink excessively—often becoming obsessed with water and eating ravenously in an attempt to quell the Fire. Their Shen, or spirit, is then disturbed, because the Heat spills over into the Heart. The Heart, which is said to house the spirit, beats faster, and eventually the cat may be diagnosed with a cardiomyopathy. A cat may be demonstrating symptoms of disturbed Heart spirit when he is anxious and begins to yowl excessively.

While holistic medicine sees hyperthyroidism as a secondary problem—more of a symptom of an underlying Yin deficiency—the conventional treatment is to destroy or remove the thyroid gland. For older cats with thyroid conditions, each of the three conventional methods for accomplishing this holds its own set of inherent dangers.

Radioactive treatment selectively radiates the thyroid gland, hastily normalizing blood pressure. This drastic lowering of blood pressure can result in kidney failure, especially in older patients with preexisting renal disease. Medication with methimazole (Tapazole) can chemically inhibit the synthesis of thyroid hormones, but it often has harmful side effects: decreased blood cells, anorexia, and weakness. Surgery, the third option, has fallen out of favor because inadvertent removal of the tiny parathyroid glands is all too common. These glands lie next to the thyroid and can be difficult to see. If these glands are removed with the thyroid, blood calcium levels become dangerously low. For younger cats, who are more resistant to side effects, radiation is often the best conventional option. There is no doubt that conventional treatments may be necessary, especially in the later stages.

There are many obvious reasons for leaving the gland intact. The idea that the thyroid gland itself is toxic is not really in agreement with a holistic view of the body. The gland is doing what it is supposed to do; it's just doing it too much. The thyroid gland is responsible for much more than just producing thyroxin; along with the parathyroid glands on either side, it has an important function in maintaining the balance of calcium in the body.

The decision to treat feline hyperthyroidism holistically boils down to a few important questions. How long has the cat been symptomatic? How old is the cat? Is he healthy otherwise? How would he take to acupuncture, herbs, or nutritional changes? Even more than other patients, hyperthyroid cats need to relax into the acupuncture treatment and allow the calming endorphins to overcome their hyperthyroid-induced anxiety.

When I first treated Mikey, I warned Trip that holistic care cannot always reverse the high thyroid hormone levels that show up on blood tests. Although acupuncture and herbs can treat the root of thyroid disease, success depends on how far along the disease has progressed and how sensitive the animal is to holistic medicine. As I petted Mikey's dry orange coat and examined where he had pulled out hair, I spoke to Trip. "Holistic medicine cannot always slow the heart rate. Sometimes conventional radioactive therapy or methimazole medication may be necessary. At the very least, holistic medicine can help enough so that the oral dose of methimazole can be lowered to safer levels or given transdermally, through the skin. This might help prevent its gastrointestinal side effects. Whether a cat needs both conventional medical treatment as well as holistic care depends on how far the disease has progressed." I could feel Mikey's heart pounding beneath his protruding ribs.

In my clinic, Trip paced like no other client, asking question after question. Finally, he asked, "Can you talk to Mikey's other vet?" He wanted to explore how much Western medicine was needed. It was a tough question, and I did not yet know, but I thought it would be better to talk to Mikey's mainstream veterinarian and just touch base.

With Trip and Mikey in the exam room, I called their regular vet. "I don't quite understand," she said flatly. "I think he has cancer and that's why he is vomiting." I thought about it. She might have been right, of course. But in Western medicine, we are trained to look for many concurrent diseases, often overlooking the fact that interrelated symptoms may share one explanation. She added, "We want to schedule an intestinal endoscopy and biopsy as soon as possible."

"Well, the methimazole could be making the cat sick." Unfortunately, even small doses of methimazole, the chemotherapylike medication used to kill thyroid cells, lowered his white and red blood cell counts to about half their normal levels. On methimazole, Mikey felt sick—he had no energy and moped around the house. "He's older and he may be more sensitive to the drug," I said. I had become accustomed to these types of conversations with conventional practitioners. I try to contact them, despite their occasional complete disbelief in what I say. It's difficult, and I have to struggle to remain open-minded to their suggestions as well.

For several minutes afterward, I listened to the regular veterinarian tell me about her experiences with intestinal cancer and how it's on the rise. I felt as if she had heard not one word I'd said.

"Trip, this decision to do a biopsy is yours. Your regular vet is convinced Mikey has cancer. I am convinced he doesn't because of one thing—he is eating ravenously. Cats with intestinal cancer are usually anorexic. I think we should do acupuncture, see how he responds, and make the decision about a biopsy in a few weeks, when he's healthier. Anesthesia would be hard on him now."

There were few viable and safe conventional options for Mikey. Trip looked at his bedraggled feline friend and agreed to bring Mikey in for weekly acupuncture treatments and herbal therapy.

"What about Mikey's urinary tract infection?" Trip asked, adjusting his eyeglasses while he resumed pacing.

I reviewed the results of Mikey's last urinalysis. No bacteria or other infectious organisms present, just red and white blood cells in the urine. In Western medicine, his urinary inflammation might be called sterile cystitis, a very frustrating thing to treat. In Chinese medicine, it was nothing more than an extension of excess Heat invading the bladder. "Let's give him an herbal tea and recheck the urine sample in ten days," I said.

Mikey watched us both. He was so wise, and I felt somehow that he would tell me what was best. Swinging his tail back and forth a little, he cried, as if to say, "Guys, make a decision. I have an appointment to keep with my dinner." One thing I have learned is that you don't want to stand between a hyperthyroid cat and his food.

First, though, I used acupuncture points to strengthen Yin, or fluids, to quell Fire, to support the kidneys and bladder. I spread the dry orange fur to find familiar points in the feet, belly, and neck. I used my tiniest thirty-eight-gauge acupuncture needles because he was so skinny and the points were very superficial. Mikey was cooperative and relaxed, as long as I stayed close. I made up an herbal combination that Trip would have to boil into a medicinal tea. It included cooling Western herbs such as yarrow to stop Blood or Heat from invading the urine, *Uva ursi* to clean the bladder wall, and plantain and marshmallow, which provide a slimy, healing coating.

The following week, I repeated the same acupuncture points. Trip said, "Mikey is yowling as if he were still hearing squirrels chasing each other through the walls and pittering around in the attic."

"It'll take several months for his hormones to balance enough to calm him down. Hyperthyroidism is thought to increase the body's sensitivity to epinephrine or adrenaline, one of the 'flight-or-fight' hormones," I said, taking out the needles.

After his urinary tract problem cleared up, I placed Mikey on Chinese herbal powder made from concentrated-extract granules. The dose would be very small—only one eighth of a teaspoon twice a day. Cats are difficult patients when it comes to administering herbs. The formula was Wei Ling Tan with the addition of two extra herbs, forsythia and rehmannia. Wei Ling Tan is a classic formula for Dampness and Heat. Forsythia cools the blood and relieves Phlegm Stagnation in the neck area, and rehmannia cools and nourishes the kidneys. On this formula and with only one acupuncture visit every six weeks or so, Mikey gained his weight back, his coat became moist and shiny, and best of all, he relaxed back into his normal self.

The final natural remedy was that the two bachelors, Trip and Mikey, moved in with Trip's girlfriend. Mikey went from visiting the neighbors to satisfy his extroverted needs to the utter bliss of life in a permanent summer camp, surrounded by children, people, and dogs. At seventeen years of age, Mikey has gained back his confidence. He lounges on sofa backs and windowsills and softly sways his draped tail as if to say, "Be one with yourself. Relax." His eyes are half closed and his lips are raised as though he is smiling.

I wish I could take full credit for his improved health, but I know how important emotions are in healing. If the owners are depressed and negative, the pet will reflect their views. If they create a loving, open space, healing will often happen with only a small nudge.

Thyroid Diseases in Cats and Dogs

The thyroid gland lies at the center of the front of the neck, where an animal's Adam's apple would be. Though such small glands, the thyroid and its neighbors on either side, the parathyroid glands, are essential for normal blood levels of calcium. The thyroid gland helps to regulate the metabolism of every cell in the body. Cats usually acquire hyperthyroidism, the opposite of dogs, whose thyroids tend to become underactive. For horses, the thyroid gland is thought to be less important in governing metabolism than the elaborate adrenaline-creating sympathetic nervous system.

The thyroid gland needs dietary iodine, but too much can be almost as detrimental as too little. Too little can cause a goiterlike condition known as hypothyroidism and too much can also have an antithyroid, or toxic, effect on hormone production. Most commercial dog and cat foods have over five times what we believe to be the necessary amount of iodine. Hypothyroidism in dogs is often easier to treat holistically than hyperthyroidism in cats. Some animals need only holistic intervention to improve, while others need a combination of holistic and conventional approaches.

CATS

Feline hyperthyroidism was not characterized in the veterinary scientific literature until 1979, which is 144 years after Robert Graves described hyperthyroidism in humans. Now it is the most commonly diagnosed endocrine condition in cats six to twelve years old. Since it is such a newly described disease in cats, we are still learning about it. Right now, it is diagnosed using a blood test that looks for both T_4 and free T_4, also called a thyroid panel, along with symptoms. The trick is to catch it early and treat it before it gets worse. Try holistic medicine! Acupuncture to resolve Dampness and strengthen the Yin, or help the body's fluids in nourishing the body's tissues, is a good first step. Indoor cats need no vaccinations; try limiting vaccines in outdoor cats, especially when they are over five years old, other than for rabies (see page 61).

Prevention is key. Go to a holistic veterinarian if you see any symptom of early disease. The well-known Canadian holistic veterinarian Dr. Steve Marsden has described many herbal combinations, depending upon the level of pathology, and these formulas are excellent for relieving symptoms. Ask your veterinarian to contact AHVMA (the American Holistic Veterinary Medical Association) for Dr. Marsden's specific recommendations.

My recommendation for feline hyperthyroidism is to try this very safe formula:

Wei Ling Tang, also called Magnolia and Hoelen Combination (2 parts)
Forsythia, also called Lian Qiao (1 part)
Rehmannia, also called Sheng di Huang (1 part)

These herbs are in concentrated-extract granule (powdered) form for a cat because less volume is needed to attain a medicinal effect and because giving herbs to cats is difficult. Give your average 10-pound cat ⅛ teaspoon twice a day in food. Perhaps after he has been on the herbs for four to six weeks, you and your veterinarian can lower his dose of methimazole (Tapazole) according to blood test results and clinical symptoms.

For aged cats in the early stages of hyperthyroidism, it may be unwise to suppress thyroxin production with methimazole because this can cause a drastic change in cardiac output, which aggravates any preexisting kidney disease. Holistic medicine can work wonders, especially for older cats. And even no treatment may be better than methimazole for elderly felines. Cats can tolerate low-grade hyperthyroidism (slightly elevated T_4 levels), with its mild hypertension, in order to promote renal perfusion and preserve kidney function. If your cat already has heart problems, please medicate him or her as directed. Propranolol has helped saved a lot of cats at this advanced level of pathology.

DOGS

When dogs are sick for almost any reason, their thyroid hormone levels may drop. A variety of drugs impair plasma or tissue binding of the thyroid hormones, including glucocorticoids, anticonvulsants, and anti-inflammatories. Anesthesia and surgery seem to alter thyroid levels in different ways depending on the drugs used.

One of the most common causes of hypothyroidism in dogs is lymphocytic thryroiditis, an immune-mediated disease caused by the animal's own white blood cells attacking his or her thyroid gland. Many veterinary immunologists, most notably Dr. Jean Dodds, consider this to be an immune-mediated disease triggered by overvaccination or other environmental exposures in genetically susceptible individuals. The many

141

symptoms may include lethargy, mental dullness, hair loss, weight gain, slow heart rate, seizures, or sudden aggression. Blood tests may show high cholesterol or anemia. A comprehensive evaluation of thyroid function and autoantibody production is the best way to diagnose this disease. Just a simple test for free T_4 is not specific enough. Animals are often unnecessarily placed on a thyroid replacement drug (thyroxin, soloxine) based on inadequate testing. Early cardiac disease may be confused with one of the most common symptoms of hypothyroidism—exercise intolerance. Most veterinarians only listen to the heart with a stethoscope, and thus cardiac disease can certainly go undiagnosed. Thyroid replacement drugs should be reserved only for those cases in which herbs, homemade food, and acupuncture cannot reverse symptoms.

Herbal Tea for Canine Hypothyroidism

4 cups low-sodium chicken broth or water
2 whole roots red Chinese ginseng (*Panax schinseng*)
¼ cup hawthorn berries
2 tablespoons ground cinnamon
2 tablespoons ground turmeric
2 teaspoons grated fresh gingerroot

Combine all of the ingredients in a small stainless steel or ceramic saucepan, cover, and simmer over low heat for 30 minutes. Remove from the heat, uncover, and let cool. Strain the tea, discarding the solids.

Keeping: The tea will last for up to 2 weeks in the refrigerator. You can also freeze it in an ice cube tray, and thaw each cube as needed. Bring to room temperature before using.

Dosing: Give 1 tablespoon per 40 pounds of body weight per day in food. This can be given for the remainder of the dog's life and is safe to use with conventional medication, but blood tests should be done regularly to see if the dose of medication needs to be altered.

THE TERRIBLE TIGER LILY

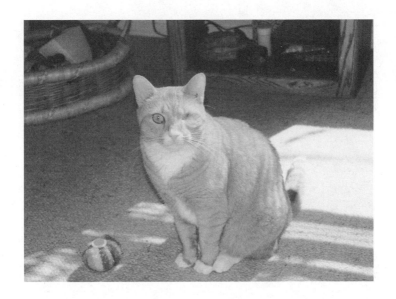

When I first met Tiger Lily on a house call in the summer of 1996, she had a lot to be grumpy about. She was a cat with a mouth full of red ulcers. She was weak from eating less and had only enough energy to be hostile. The orange tabby had been sick for several years. Anna and Spike, her cat mates, lived in fear of Tiger's increasingly frequent attacks; she released her wrath by hissing, growling, and even batting their heads as they tried to sleep. Her human, Jackie Bergmann, and I stood on opposite sides of a makeshift exam table in the center of Jackie's kitchen. We contemplated the fate of Tiger Lily who, had she been any other cat, would have given up on life months earlier.

The feisty orange tabby sat before us curled in a protective ball, ears flat back against her head, peering at me from her one remaining eye. Like a weathered pirate, Tiger had only a crevasse where her left eye had been. She wrapped her tail tightly around her tense body, like a scared old lady clutching her handbag. There was something compelling about her demeanor. She was tough, and I admired her for that. At times, as one of the only holistic vets in Seattle, I wish I could be as strong as Tiger in the face of criticism and judgment about my work.

I glanced at the small orange cat and she hissed disapproval so explicit in its intent that I shuddered and backed away. If she wouldn't let me look at her, how could I ever do acupuncture on her? Could all this anger result from pain? Inside the open hissing mouth I saw the problem—big, red, ulcerated lesions on both sides of Tiger's mouth, like hot, erupting volcanoes, on the side pillars connecting the upper and lower jaws.

As if Jackie had bionic X-ray vision, she could see a kind cat behind all that anger. Where the rest of the world saw the growling and hissing as signs to stay away, Jackie viewed them as a cry for help and reached out even further to Tiger. She loved the one-eyed feline more than any other animal she had ever known. When Tiger hid from her, Jackie got motivated to find a cure for the cat's pain.

According to Jackie, when she first met the homeless, declawed street cat, both of them were living in Weehawken, New Jersey. Tiger was no stranger to the pains of the real world. Showing every bone in her body, Tiger found a friend in Jackie, and trusted her enough to cry for food. In the shadows of the Weehawken buildings, Tiger had made do. How did the world seem to this orange sack of skin and bones? I picture her back then as Jackie described her: whiskers at half-mast, black tar and stains tarnishing her orange coat.

Once they moved to Seattle, Tiger Lily became infamous at the local veterinary hospital. There she received her nickname "terrible" by screaming at the top of her feline lungs in the back treatment room, sending a collective chill down the spines of other clients. After every examination, a ruffled veterinary technician would emerge with the equally frazzled Tiger Lily in a carrier, both of them breathless and frightened from the encounter. If the gossip about Tiger was true, a bite from the terrible Tiger Lily was an expected occupational hazard.

Although Tiger was no fan of veterinarians, she had certainly met her share of them. And they remembered her the way you remember the bully at recess. Tiger's disfigured eye was removed, but after complications, two surgeries were needed. Tiger was diagnosed with a heart murmur, early kidney disease, and ulcers in her mouth, which had since gotten worse. Jackie was shown the pathology report after oral biopsies were taken: "Lymphocytic, plasmacytic stomatitis," it said, which basically meant an inflammatory process affecting the tissues of her mouth. While she was under anesthesia for dentistry, the veterinarian removed the ulcerated mouth nodules, and even though this surgery was repeated, the ulcers returned. For three years, Tiger had steroid shots every few weeks to suppress her stomatitis, and as a result she then developed a transient form of diabetes. Now the only form of conventional treatment offered to Tiger, steroids to suppress the immune system, had become too risky.

If there was ever a dead-end disease in Western medicine, this was it. When pushed for an explanation, conventional veterinarians could only loosely relate the stomatitis to a variety of underlying causes, such as an accumulation of dental tartar, bacteria, viral infection, and genetic predisposition. The conventional treatment was to extract all the teeth in an attempt to remove the source of dental bacteria, followed by steroid pills to suppress the body's severe immune system reaction. That explanation and treatment did not sit well with me. Why would some cats and not others exhibit such inflammation when the amount of dental tartar and bacteria was similar? Even if all their teeth are pulled, many cats continue to be riddled with the disease.

The condition can be better explained from a holistic Chinese medical perspective. There are a few factors that, given a certain body constitution, result in this disease. As with other immune-mediated diseases, too many vaccines might cause the immune system to overreact so that even normal oral bacteria will trigger an inflammatory response.

Individual constitutional differences explain why some cats acquire this autoimmune disease and others do not. There is a congenital constitution that incorporates genetic weakness, which comes with purebred, especially inbred, animals. An acquired constitution takes into consideration other factors since birth, such as the vaccination and medication history, the input of the animal's owner, and the cat's emotional sensitivities. In my experience, many cats with stomatitis have had very difficult histories. They may develop angry Liver, which often causes pain and results in aggressive behavior.

Commercial cat food can aggravate mouth inflammation because dry cat food is coated with fat to make it more appetizing. Dry kibble is energetically hot and dry. It lacks moisture, and the fat content generates Heat. It depletes the body's fluids and Yin. The Kidney is the source of all Yin energy in the body, and over time this Kidney Yin becomes depleted. The teeth are an extension of the bones, and the Kidney governs the bones.

Without the cooling and moistening properties of enough fluid, Heat builds up in the body and the tissues dry out. Specific meridians that course through the mouth tend to accumulate this Heat. They are the internal branches of the Large Intestine, Stomach, and Liver. This explains the Chinese medical diagnosis of Stomach or Liver Fire. This heat causes redness, inflammation, bleeding, and pain.

About the feline diet—cats evolved while eating mice! They were supposed to keep their teeth clean by crunching on raw mouse bones and get vegetable matter from the mouse intestines and from grazing on grass. Mice contain a lot more natural water content than does dry cat food, which is why in nature cats don't need to drink as much. Switching to soft or canned foods can help stomatitis.

Most of the cats with stomatitis eat less, because food irritates the mouth ulcers. But I have found that cats like Tiger, who have truly known starvation, will not stop eating unless they are almost at death's doorstep. Stomach Fire also causes excess hunger. We could tell that eating was very painful because afterward, Tiger would violently paw and swipe at her mouth, circling, spinning, and backing into corners. Ricocheting off furniture became a daily event that followed each meal.

Most people probably would have given up on such a difficult and diseased cat. Tiger was mean and dangerous and had no inhibitions about shredding your arm. But Jackie is an unusually compassionate champion of animals. She told me, "I like the animals other people ignore." It seemed true. She befriends crows, homeless cats, and the odd seagull.

She is the type of person who would think nothing of rushing into a burning building to rescue an animal, even if her own life were at risk. She is six feet tall and has short wispy brown hair; her dark blue eyes gaze upon her animals with the tender concern of a parent. The scabs on Jackie's hands were from Tiger, but Jackie didn't hold that against her cat, justifying her wounds as products of the cat's fear. In fact, she recited the cause for each injury as if she were showing me a photo album: "Oh, this big one on my thumb was from our airplane trip from New Jersey . . . and this one on my pinkie was after the most recent blood draw." Jackie was so proud of the street cat she had once saved.

We pondered our next course of action. "Well, at least she's weakened by the diabetes. Maybe she won't bite as hard," Jackie said, smiling a little. Normally when I acupuncture cats, I lift their feet and position their bodies to insert the needles into the correct points, but Tiger would be difficult to touch.

"Let's try something. If we have a way to move her on the table without touching her, it might be safer," I said. The orange cat hissed again, as if she were part of the conversation. Her hiss was not like the usual superficial gesture of most house cats but was more like what you might hear at the zoo when standing in front of a real jungle tiger. Tiger's hisses were guttural, using all of her extra lung space for emphasis.

Although the fabric might not have been Tiger's first choice, we found a pink flannel cat-print blanket. By placing the blanket on our slippery counter/exam table, we could rotate Tiger on top instead of picking her up to turn her. Jackie and I would eventually come to refer to her treatments as "spinning."

On that summer Wednesday in July 1996, I inserted small Chinese needles in each point—I chose points to quench Stomach and Liver Fire on each back toe, and to support Kidney function right above where the kidneys are located. Tiger turned to warn me, but I proceeded cautiously and she never actually snapped at me.

After a while, Jackie lifted Tiger's front feet, allowing me to needle important, difficult-to-reach points in between Tiger's back legs, like Stomach 44, which clears Stomach Fire; Kidney 7, which moistens Dryness and supports Yin; and Bladder 39, which regulates the Triple Heater and resolves Damp Heat.

Acupuncture points have beautiful Chinese names too that relate to their anatomical location or function—Stomach 44 is also "inner courtyard," and Kidney 7 is otherwise known as "repeated current," which refers to its ability to regulate body fluids. Spleen 6 is "three-Yin junction," a point that tonifies the Spleen and Yin of the body. In Chinese medicine, the Spleen shares the pancreatic function of transforming food into Qi. Spleen 6 reduces digestive stagnation and clears Fire due to Yin deficiency. Since the pancreas produces insulin, this point was particularly important.

Like tiny messengers, the Chinese needles work by stimulating nerves that go to the spinal cord and tell the organs of the body to perform better. They redirected the inflammation, or hot fire, from Tiger's mouth to where the needle entered the body, similar to what happens when you prick yourself accidentally. The difference is that this action is directed at a specific point in a specific way that restores the smooth flow of Qi, or life's energy, to a stagnant area along the meridians. The needles are so small and feline skin so flexible, cats rarely feel them. A sedating or endorphin-induced effect takes place, and cats close their eyes and rest.

Jackie was right; Tiger Lily didn't fight the needles. In fact, once they were in, she seemed quite content, staring glazed-eyed toward a fixed point in the middle of the room. Judging from her wide pupils, deep breathing, and stillness, I knew the endorphins were acting on her debilitated body. She relaxed a little but still hissed skeptically if I moved too suddenly.

"How long have you and Tiger lived here in Seattle?" I asked, gently rotating the cat's needles to stimulate them.

"About six years. She didn't like the plane trip, and it was tough for her to adapt to living inside. Lately I've wondered if I did the right thing in bringing her to Washington. Ever since we got here, she's been so sick."

Jackie resumed stroking the cat's whiskers and chest. "Maybe she is really no better off," she added. Knowing the urban nature of Weehawken after having lived in New Jersey, I thought that Jackie's statement was a little extreme. But she was not joking; her eyes misted with compassion.

"We'll know in just a few treatments," I answered. But honestly, I knew it would be tough going. We needed to pull her through this crisis and help heal her mouth all at once. I worried that as soon as Tiger felt better, maybe she wouldn't let me treat her again. If she really was a mean cat, and not just sick, maybe acupuncture every week was wishful thinking on my part.

Jackie's cat clock on the wall ticked rhythmically, and its pendulum tail swung back and forth. Jackie and I were suspended in a state of unknowing calm, observing the patient. Tiger Lily's famous temperamental personality seemed to transform right under our eyes. At this particular moment, attacking me was the farthest thing from her mind. Where her body had been fearful, crouching, and tense, she was now relaxed, eye at half-mast, her pain lifting.

I looked around at Jackie's house, which she had bought with the cats in mind. "You never know when a landlord might get tired of animals and kick you out," she remarked. I knew Jackie was a lot like Tiger Lily; the world had always been a little harsh, a little unpredictable to her. In looking for a house, most people would imagine the placement of a favorite couch or love seat, but Jackie envisioned her cats' favorite furniture: scratching posts, climbing trees, and a bay window for catnaps in the sun.

Other things in Jackie's house looked as if they tended to get ignored in favor of animal care. The bills, papers, and lists that normally would occupy a kitchen counter were tossed aside, replaced by a wicker basket of Tiger's medications. Pictures, knickknacks, and the bric-a-brac of cat dishes and crow statues cluttered the shelves. Fake tiger-skin furniture covers adorned the couch.

In addition to weekly acupuncture, I prescribed a homemade diet, vitamins, and herbs. Afterward Jackie reported that as I had guessed, Tiger Lily was less than cooperative about a change in her food. She refused to tolerate any newfangled homemade diets. Having become accustomed to the fat-coated Hill's K/D, she wouldn't even sniff some of Jackie's best cooking. The menu could have come from New York's fanciest restaurants: mackerel and squash, organic chicken and couscous, cod and quinoa. I usually try different foods, and if a cat seems interested, I recommend adding vitamins and small amounts of other meats, the way an artist might build a sculpture.

Homemade gourmet diets were definitely rejected not just by Tiger but by Anna and Spike too. Jackie told me, "I spent seventy dollars on all that weird food. The cats wouldn't eat it and broke into one of my cabinets and opened a tin of dog biscuits I keep for the neighbor's dog. I came home from work to little pieces of gnawed-on Milk-Bones. It was a sign that health food was definitely out. I even tried cod liver oil, because the pet store said that might entice them. Afterward, the cats wouldn't even set foot in the kitchen. They were offended by the smell!"

Between us, Jackie and I tried practically every way of improving Tiger's nutrition, but to no avail—until one day, Jackie opened a jar of baby food, organic peas and rice. With four other dishes on the kitchen floor in front of her, Tiger went for the vegetarian baby food! Next we added some vitamins and other supplements, and Tiger ate all of it along with the original commercial cat food. Since she couldn't kick the K/D habit, we decided not to fight her. We thought her days were numbered.

After the first treatment, Jackie noticed that Tiger was feeling better because she stopped hiding in dark corners. Instead of attacking her housemates, she slept with Anna, a beautiful black shelter-rescued cat, in the sun window and playfully pawed at Spike, another large orange tabby, as he walked by. Spike always reminded me of Norm on *Cheers* because of his satirical smirk.

At night, when the rain fell softly in the chilly Seattle winter, Jackie told me that Tiger started to show the tender side she had always known was there. The cat would jump onto Jackie's bed, purr as loudly as a motorcar, and want to be held like a teddy bear. To Jackie, Tiger's purr and her cuddly nature felt like a sip of Grandma's hot cocoa. Of all three cats, Tiger was the one most in tune with Jackie's emotions. If Jackie had a bad day at work, Tiger knew it right away and purred louder to make up for it.

Although she still hissed when I came around, the new and improved, adventurous Tiger Lily became the first to explore new kitty litter, introduce herself to the new goldfish, and jump onto the bed next to Jackie at night. While Tiger still had swiping fits, they were less frequent and less severe. Her transient diabetes had disappeared fast. She did not need insulin shots. Her blood glucose returned to normal, which might have happened just because an alternative to steroid therapy was used. Best of all, Tiger Lily became nicer than Jackie had ever known her to be.

Tiger endured weekly acupuncture for two months, during which time Jackie happily reported an improvement in her personality. She even softened some toward me. Although we still used the blanket spin method, Tiger relaxed her clamped body, stopped hissing, and regarded me with a normal ear stance instead of holding them pressed hard against her scalp, ready to pounce.

But what about those nasty mouth volcanoes and lava beds? When we looked inside Tiger's mouth, they were still there, but less inflamed and causing fewer painful episodes. Over time, Jackie learned whether the mouth ulcers were flaring up from Tiger's behavior. If Tiger was in a little pain, she would wipe her tongue from side to side. If she was in more pain, she would swipe angrily at her mouth with both paws at once. But the violent pawing episodes were gone.

I taught Jackie to do acupressure between visits, using a modified T-touch on the most important acupuncture points. With a soft, clockwise massage method, Jackie pressed Kidney and Governing Vessel points, the most important one Governing Vessel 20. Thought to release the most pain-relieving endorphins, it is located right on top of the head. Like the acupuncture, acupressure alleviated Tiger's mouth pain by diverting painful impulses, much the way you would kick a soccer ball away if you were a goalie. Over the following weeks, I started decreasing the number of acupuncture treatments to once every few weeks. "I did Tiger's Governing Vessel," Jackie said when I saw her, smiling at the foreign-sounding ring of it.

After about six months, the symptoms of Tiger's stomatitis seemed to have vanished. Every time Tiger looked a little out of sorts, had ruffled fur, or ate a little less—which amounted to every two to three weeks—Jackie called me for another acupuncture spin session. Tiger was steroid, vaccine, and conventional-medicine free from her first treatment on. She developed a few new problems over the years, such as ear discharge (Liver disharmony) and joint pain (Kidney imbalance). I changed my point locations for Tiger over time, and in her later years cleaned her ears out, which was more stressful than acupuncture.

About the time I started treating Tiger, I had a puppy come into the emergency room at two in the morning. Over the years of doing animal emergency room work, I had to shut off emotionally in order to cope with the sad things I saw—dogs hit by cars, or a warmth-seeking cat who had been trapped in a car's fan belt. Two young women brought in a shepherd

puppy who had obviously suffered a terrible fracture of his front leg. He hobbled in, and a small boy trailed behind. I noticed a big man waiting outside the front door, but I thought nothing of it. After examining the puppy, I asked how the accident had happened, since there were no external abrasions or cuts as there usually are when a dog is hit by a car. The women looked at one another, shrugged, and said, "We don't know." One of them shifted a little. "We don't have any money anyway," she said.

"Well, a puppy can't just break its leg," I said. The boy began aggressively pulling on the puppy's tail; the women didn't seem to notice. They shrugged again. "I can take your dog, find him a good home, and fix the leg," I said, but they would hear nothing of it and flatly refused.

I told the boy that his puppy was in pain and not to torment him. I took the puppy into the back treatment area and said a little prayer for him while I applied a splint to his leg. The women never did reveal what had really happened. I gave them some phone numbers of vets who might work on a sliding scale and might fix the fracture the next day. I was upset because I suspected abuse but was afraid because I was alone at the hospital in the middle of the night.

Suddenly the man stormed in and grabbed the puppy. "Come on," he barked at the women. "I'm takin' this piece-of-shit dog home." The man threatened me and left, slamming the door behind him. The women and the boy followed, and I locked the door behind them and called the police in case they returned. I was wide-eyed and trembling the rest of the night.

Some nights later, I dreamed that instead of letting the puppy go, I followed behind, yelling at the man, ordering him to give me the puppy. In my dream, I was angry and afraid, and like Tiger Lily, perhaps, those emotions propelled my actions. Like a coiled tigress, I pounced on the man and told him to pick on someone his own size. I was as strong as a superhero, as courageous as a stray orange cat left without claws to defend herself in Weehawken. If I were ever threatened again, I could call upon Tiger as a role model to give me courage. I certainly would always remember hers.

Slowly, Tiger Lily transformed from a ferocious to a friendly feline. I remember the first time I noticed Tiger actually accepting me. On a Sunday morning about six months after we started treatments, I drove to Jackie's house and saw her on the front lawn, ambling between the

peonies and the birdbath. She was still in her robe and slippers. She threw handful after handful of peanuts to an accumulating flock of crows gathered there for brunch. I sat in my car watching the birds nearly taking the nuts from her hands and Jackie speaking to them as if she knew them all by name. And being the talkative birds that crows are, unfortunately for the neighbors, they cawed back.

"Good morning," she said when she saw me. "Tiger is looking forward to her treatment." Jackie always said that, and I had never believed her. But this time, when we entered the house, Tiger Lily was the first one to greet me at the door. Her orange body rubbed up against my shins; her tail wrapped around my ankles like a tiny python. Her purr was as loud as rumbles of thunder disappearing into the distance after a storm.

"Wow. Has Tiger become a sweet kitty lately?" I asked in astonishment.

"Tiger's been trying to thank you all along, but you were too busy to notice," Jackie answered, rearranging her seagull statue to face the street. We did the treatment that week without the blanket. It is clear to me now that Tiger's aggression was, as Jackie had always insisted, just a result of her pain.

When cats hiss at me now, I consider whether it is pain causing their outbursts. It makes me more sympathetic toward what they feel. That day, I heard Tiger's purr loud in the chill of the autumn morning. If she could speak, I'm sure she would have said, "Never show your weakness."

Tiger Lily had more than six healthy, wonderful years with Jackie. The mouth problem that almost cost her her life eventually went away. When she died of kidney failure, I realized there was no cat patient I'd miss more than Tiger. I cried with Jackie, and I knew I would always remember the tenacious spunk of the one-eyed Tiger Lily from Weehawken.

Mouth Problems in Pets

Problems in pets' mouths are easy to miss for one reason: The mouth is difficult to examine and we rarely get a good look inside. If you get your pet used to oral exams from an early age, life will be easier, believe it or not, on him or her and on your veterinarian. According to traditional Chi-

nese medicine, the Stomach, Liver, and Large Intestine meridians run right through the mouth. Therefore, a healthy mouth and good-smelling breath often reflect a healthy digestive system. Many commercial pet foods give animals bad breath, or halitosis, while homemade foods leave the mouth smelling fresh.

You might be able to tell that there is something wrong with the gums, teeth, or mouth if the animal will not eat at all, eats less than normal, or seems uncomfortable when he or she eats. Other symptoms include bad-smelling breath, bleeding, swelling or redness around gums or cheeks, and unexplained listlessness.

HOW TO EXAMINE YOUR PET'S MOUTH

Put your pet on a table or on the floor and position yourself behind him or her. Slip your fingers under his lips and just look at the gums on both the right and the left. You do not need to pry the mouth open. The teeth should be white and the gums uniformly pink. Are the gums red around the tooth roots? Is there plaque or brown tartar on the teeth? (If you have a cat or a dog, be happy, because a full-mouth speculum has to be used on horses to know what is going on in their mouths!) Look for abnormal growths and show your veterinarian. Regular oral exams are one of the most important reasons to go to your vet.

TREATMENT FOR COMMON MOUTH PROBLEMS

If there is severe gum redness or yellow or brown tartar buildup on teeth, take your pet in for a dental cleaning. Oftentimes, dental problems are too bad to manage at home. I have seen cats and dogs experience new energy after dental work because, after I clean or remove loose teeth, the animal is no longer in pain. But dogs and cats require anesthesia to clean their teeth, which has its own set of risks. Preventive care should start at the puppy or kitten stage if only to get your pet accustomed to brushing.

Gingivitis is extremely common in cats and certain breeds of dogs—dachshunds, greyhounds, small poodles, Malteses. It might have something to do with genetics and salivary enzymes, but I have seen homemade diets, especially those including raw beef knuckle bones, chicken necks, and turkey backs, clean very dirty teeth without any brushing. Poor cats—if only they chewed on mice, they could brush their own teeth! They suffer so much with bleeding and red or painful gums. Brush their teeth (just brush the outside—no need to open the mouth) with a child's soft-bristled toothbrush. Finger toothbrushes don't work if tartar is present. Poultry-flavored toothpaste is very helpful even if it's used only three times a week. In addition to brushing, feeding the powerful antioxidant coenzyme Q_{10}, 30 milligrams for an average cat and 90 milligrams for a 50-pound dog, will help promote healing and circulation in the gums. Just open the capsule into your pet's food.

Stomatitis is a very serious autoimmune disease. It differs from gingivitis in that the red inflammation is not only around the teeth but is in a much larger area, including the upper and/or lower back of the mouth. Cats suffer extreme pain during and after eating, or may choose not to eat. Holistic veterinarians can offer alternatives to steroid therapy. If you are in an area with no holistic vets, try the following formula for minor stomatitis: 2 teaspoons warm water or chicken broth, ½ teaspoon honey, ¼ teaspoon slippery elm bark powder, 1 drop clove oil. One cc or milliliter of this mixture can be applied safely to inflamed gums with a three-milliliter syringe once or twice a day.

For more severe stomatitis, as diagnosed by your veterinarian, try the following herbal recipe. These are Northwest herbs used in tincture form:

Redroot (*Ceanothus velutinus*), 2 parts. Not to be confused with blood-
   root.
Spilanthes, 1 part
Gromwell (*Lithospermum rudale*), 1 part
Betony (*Pedicularis racemosa*), 1 part

Ceanothus is used to regulate immune-system function and to drain lymphatic blockage; *Spilanthes* is used by Northwest Native Americans for toothaches and to relieve pain; *Lithospermum* is used in immune-mediated disease; and *Pedicularis* is used to treat pain and inflammation, especially of the head.

Usually, I do not recommend any alcohol-based herbal treatments for cats and dogs, but because it is difficult to orally medicate a cat with stomatitis, this tincture works well because the kitty needs only 4 to 6 drops a day.

Wrap the cat in a towel and, as always, stand behind the animal when giving oral medications, especially if your pet is tough to treat.

Tartar formation is very common even if your pet eats kibble. Eating kibble does not prevent tartar. Tartar can form more quickly after numerous dental cleanings, because microscopic damage to the enamel means that the tooth loses its natural protective barriers. To avoid the cost of professional dental cleaning and anesthetic risk, take care of your pet's teeth as you would your own. Regular brushing, as well as feeding small pieces of raw chicken or turkey bones, necks, or backs for cats and raw frozen beef knuckle bones for dogs, will keep the teeth white and the gums healthy.

Bad breath is also very common. Gingivitis is the main cause. A homemade diet (pages 28–30) and even brushing the teeth with human natural fennel-flavored, or CET mint animal toothpaste, offer good prevention. Don't use traditional human toothpastes, because the frothing agents can cause gastritis. Adding a small amount of alfalfa or chlorophyll powder (⅛ teaspoon for a cat or 1 teaspoon for a 50-pound dog) to food will help too. Wheat or cat grass is another source of natural chlorophyll, and cats will normally help themselves.

Animals benefit from preventive dental care, as well as occasional professional cleanings if they become necessary. Today, there are veterinarians who specialize in dentistry, cavity filling, root canals, and even braces.

ANGEL

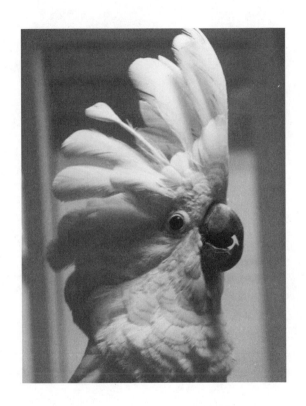

When I was a young girl, my grandfather Paul and I took long walks in the woods. He knew every type of bird, not only by its color but also by its unique call, and when we walked, he mimicked their high-pitched whistles or low coo-coos perfectly. Birds came to him; yellow finches flittered close and calico chickadees lined bushes to greet us along the trail. When his health declined, and just before he joined the bird spirits that were circling his hospital room, he told me a story that I had forgotten for many years—until one day when I met a cockatoo named Angel.

A long time ago, guardian angels and fairies chose birds to help them solve a big problem. The angels saw that above all creatures, birds could float between the spirit world and earth. The head guardian angel addressed the birds, opening her huge white feathered wings as she spoke to representatives from each of the bird species. Eagle, Barn Owl, Swallow, Duck, Toucan, Cockatoo, and Canary were among the crowd in the gleam of the sunlight. Their feathers reflected every known color. "We have watched you over many millennia and have seen that you birds, above all the other animals, have a deep altruistic capacity to love and respect all beings," she said. For a rare moment, the birds were silent. "Will you help us guide the humans away from trouble and help them connect spiritually with their world? We cannot watch over them anymore, and we fear they will destroy the place that gives them life."

When Eagle spoke, his voice reverberated throughout the canyon. "We would help, but many of us have been harmed by humans. They killed some of my own ancestors."

Barn Owl chimed in, "Humans build electric wires in my flight paths." He spun his head clear 'round to make sure the others listened. "Many of us get electrocuted. Why should we protect them?"

For more than two hundred years, humans had imprisoned Canary for no crime. He sang, "And they took us from the jungle and put us in small cages." Cockatoo agreed, as she did not like cages either, and she knew that other parrots from all corners of the world were being captured to become pets.

Toucan chimed in, and the others stared at his overgrown beak, focusing on his every word. His rainbow coloring glimmered as he spoke. "The humans destroy more of our ancient forests by the day to make way for beef cattle."

Red-tailed Hawk's dark eyes were piercing. "And paved where my forests and farms used to be." His keen sense of smell detected crude oil and tar lingering where humans had been.

Swallow's small, rapid voice peeped from the back of the room: "The humans catch us in nets."

"And shoot us with their high-powered rifles," Duck quacked.

The guardian spoke in a slow, tired tone. "We know, for we have followed humans throughout their history. We believe we can help guide them away from cruelty and toward compassion. They once hunted humpback whales, whose very song is the ancestral pulse, the spiritual thread connecting all oceans. Now humans fight for Whale's protection. And some humans have prohibited the capture of wild birds."

The birds cackled, cooed, cawed, and peeped all at once as they discussed the guardian's question. Suddenly, a tiny form flitted to the great angel. It was Green Hummingbird, who was always the first to do anything. More than the others, she understood the haste with which a lifetime passes. "I will remind humans that the world is theirs only temporarily and that they should preserve the planet for the next incarnations. When they see me, they will feel as if they were touched by a fairy from the spirit world."

Cockatoo, being especially emotionally and spiritually aware, knew she would be of particular use. "Who could better understand humans than we parrots? Many of us live day to day with them. We can try to nudge them toward better choices."

One by one, the others followed in agreement. The guardian gave them this mission: "You will need to appear to the most despairing humans, those who have truly lost their way, and give them heart and courage."

Months before I met Angel, Dr. Tracy Bennett had been struck by the bird's kind and generous personality and told me stories about the cockatoo. She told me about Angel's powers of empathy, especially with her owner, Chris. When a family dog died, Chris was devastated, and her beautiful white cockatoo mutilated herself in despair, pulling on the paper-thin skin around her ankles. Later, Angel deliberately began doing things to cheer Chris up. Angel ate her food, which always delighted Chris, and hung upside down doing her famous "bat girl" trick.

Angel sucked her talon when she was nervous and liked to be cradled on her back like an infant. When Chris force-fed her, unlike most animals, Angel could not have been happier. She lay on her back wrapped in a little towel and softly chirped high-pitched squeaks, exactly like a baby bird being fed by its mother. While Chris read at night, Angel spent hours on Chris's forearm lovingly staring at her, as if to say, "Our time together is magical."

From the start, Angel wasn't very active or particularly fond of eating, but Chris didn't know if that was normal for her. Angel exhibited no overt symptoms of illness. Still, after a few months, Chris insisted to Tracy, in her sweet but determined manner, that Angel was sick. "I just can't describe it, but she's not quite well," Chris said, softly stroking Angel's bright white plumage.

Knowing that more than any other animals, birds hide their illnesses, Tracy ran the first blood tests of many to come. Sure enough, later that day, Tracy diagnosed Angel's underactive immune system. The cockatoo's white blood cell count was only four thousand instead of the normal ten thousand. If her white blood cells continued to drop, Angel might die from an opportunistic infection.

One by one, Angel's symptoms did appear, just as Chris had predicted they might. It was as if they were the evil characters who came to her through clairvoyant dreams: Regurgitation. Diarrhea. Fluffed feathers. Anorexia. Each morning brought a new symptom and soon Angel was depressed.

Even on antibiotics combined with other conventional care, Angel's health deteriorated over the weeks that followed. The worst symptoms were sluggish digestion and air sacculitis, a kind of bird pneumonia. Her white blood cell count dropped to three thousand. Angel's crop stopped emptying normally, and even several hours after eating, a large bolus of food sat undigested. She did not want to eat, so when her crop finally emptied, Chris fed her with a syringe.

Angel's air sacculitis also got worse. Tracy said, "We do blood tests every few weeks; radiographs show some scarring of the air sacs, and now Chris has her on a nebulizer twice a day."

How do you nebulize a bird? I wondered. Tracy's skill with her avian patients never ceased to amaze me. Later Chris showed me how she had converted her pet carrier into a vacuum-sealed oxygen chamber and plugged tubes from the nebulizing unit into the holes in the side of the carrier. Angel would sit in the makeshift medicated chamber, breathing in a fine antibiotic mist. Chris said it helped her breathe better for some time afterward. Chris treated Angel this way, in addition to giving her many other oral medications, for a few months before she came to see me. Finally, Tracy agreed to bring Chris and Angel into my clinic. She knew there was no safe form of conventional medicine that could increase Angel's white blood cell count.

Tracy and Chris brought the fading cockatoo one afternoon. Angel sat dull winged and droopy eyed on my soft-covered exam table. There was something so otherworldly about birds, and Angel was a supreme example. She is a lovely white cockatoo with sunlight yellow under each wing and summer-sky light blue circles around her dark eyes. We looked at one another with a mutual sense of intrigue. It was as if we had somehow known each other already.

"All viral tests are negative. I think she has a bacterial infection because her immune system is so weak," Tracy said, grounding me in my medical world. She wrapped Angel in a towel to prepare her for acupuncture.

I searched Angel's gaze for an answer to the obvious question—why is this young bird so sick? I wished animals could just tell me how they felt. In the case of birds, veterinarians have to take their super sleuthing to the highest level, because birds maintain their wild nature and don't like to show symptoms.

I began to think about the cockatoo's tiny body according to the principles of traditional Chinese medicine. If her Liver had been weak, she might have had more skin and eye problems. Especially given her youth, I could see that many of her problems originated in the Kidneys, which warm and moisten various body tissues. The essence or "prenatal Jing" is the vitality we are born with and is stored in the Kidneys. The "postnatal Jing" is the acquired essence we attain through proper nutrition, exercise, loving touch, and positive outlook. Prenatal Jing may roughly correlate with genetic or inherited strength and can explain why some individuals always seem sick, while others are healthy. The Kidney essence is needed to nourish the Spleen, Lung, and Bone Marrow. All of Angel's symptoms could be due to this loss of vital Essence and Jing, because the Spleen controls crop emptying, the Lung controls the air sacs, and her low white cell count originates in the Marrow.

I used tiny Korean hand needles that were easy to lose in all those white feathers. Luckily, all acupuncture needles have one tightly coiled end that prohibits them from entering the body too deeply. Chris carefully placed Angel on her back—the bird liked this, oddly enough, because she was still a baby at heart. Angel looked at me suspiciously at first, but she was so weak that acupuncture didn't faze her. No matter what species of animal I have treated, after a while the points themselves have become like old friends—I can count on them to restore health.

I decided to start in the easiest place, Angel's legs, because they are so much like dogs' legs. "Kidney three," I said aloud, placing the tiny needles amid the parted feathers on the inside of both ankle joints. It was the source point for the Kidneys and could strengthen them most effectively. Angel nibbled lovingly on Chris's finger. "Stomach thirty-six is the strongest energy-producing point in the body and Chinese studies have shown that needling it increases white blood cells," I remarked while finding the point below each knee. I chose Lung 7 on each wing to support the Lung. Angel resembled a feathered pincushion, but remained resting on her back.

The needles remained in for ten minutes. Many bird acupuncturists say birds rarely tolerate acupuncture needles for any length of time, and use only an "in-and-out" immediate release technique. Angel stood up all at once, gave one sharp flick of her feathers, and most of the needles popped out and onto the floor. Then she carefully lifted each wing and cleverly hung her head to inspect each point, making sure that I had removed the needles.

I *felt* something strange during Angel's acupuncture treatment. Through the acupuncture needles, I could feel the tingling and warmth that normally is felt by the patient spread from my fingers into my whole body. It was almost as if Angel were reaching out, attempting to touch me.

I wanted to prescribe herbs for Angel's sluggish digestion and depressed immune system. For thousands of years, herbalists on every continent have been using "energetic herbalism." In this system, a patient's constitution is balanced. If a person has a viral cold and he tends to be a cold person, an excellent treatment might be a warming herb such as raw garlic, or ginger-lime tea. If the person has a viral cold but is generally overheated, a good treatment might include cooler herbs like echinacea or goldenseal. I needed to find the system that could best describe Angel's constitution. Birds are normally hot, but Angel was cooler and drier than normal. Birds are normally fast moving, but Angel was sluggish.

I think it is impossible to address bird diseases, in general, without considering emotions. Fear attacks the Kidney and excess worry aggravates the Spleen. Owing to their flock mentality, birds have an eerie sense of their person's emotional state. Being caged also causes depression, for a bird is the ultimate embodiment of the Ayurvedic body type, vata. Vata people and animals must constantly be moving, or flying, and are most associated with air. Lack of exercise causes stagnation in energy flow. Of all domesticated birds, cockatoos are probably the most emotional, and Angel was no exception.

I used the Chinese patent formulation Gui Pi San, which I mixed with water and two single Chinese herbs, rehmannia and astragalus. Dr. David McCluggage, a well-known holistic avian veterinarian, taught me about Gui Pi San, which is also known as "Wake-the-Spleen Pills." It is used for overworked, anxious patients whose mental preoccupation has caused digestive imbalances. Adding rehmannia, I hoped, would help the Kidney and moisten Angel's body. Astragalus is a classic warm formula that slowly strengthens immune function. And Gui Pi San would build up her blood and nourish the organs.

At first, Angel improved according to plan. Weekly acupuncture and the herbal formula increased her white blood cell count from three thousand to nine thousand in only two months. For a while, instead of being a depressed bird showing no personality, she started rocking to the oldies again, her favorite music. If she saw Chris, she knocked on the window-pane with her beak. She danced-bobbed as if she were a Broadway act, hanging upside down and flapping her wings, which Chris had never seen her do before. Grabbing the steel bars on her large cage, she slid down and then used her beak like a third foot to pull herself up again.

Angel was doing so well, we decided to do just acupuncture every few weeks. But after three months, she took a nosedive. Almost overnight, Angel was back to her half-fluffed depressed ways in the corner of her cage. Chris knew the results of her blood test before they came back—Angel's white cell count had dropped to four thousand. Again, she stopped eating.

My heart sank. Just when I'd thought her body had found its own balance, Angel was in trouble again. I knew I needed to change the herbs. Something told me that if only I understood the plant medicine on a deeper spiritual level, a stronger healing could occur. I remembered how, on hikes through the Northwest forests, my grandfather had taught me to walk in the forest according to his Indian teachers. I walked softly along deforested ridges and brush-torn pathways and saw European invaders such as mullein, yarrow, and plantain. Many of these powerful healers we routinely mistake for weeds. We even poison these powerful allies, like the famous liver strengthener dandelion, while our ancestors included them in salads and brewed them for medicine.

Early one Sunday morning after learning that Angel was desperately sick again, I walked in my herb garden with the goal of listening to plant spirits. I had been taking small workshops on plant consciousness and their connection with the spirit world and had sworn for months that it could not be true—how could plants *know* more than people?

Once, after such a workshop at the Northwest Herbal Faire at the Riverfarm, near Bellingham, I found myself with a small group of herbalists. The subject was intriguing: "Healing with Plant Spirits on the Fourth Dimension." I decided to check it out. Our teacher spoke of the sucking doctors in his Native American tradition who literally sucked bad spirits out of people. He spoke of other far-out subjects, like communicating with fairies and nonconscious reality. He spoke of seeing the bright blue light of devas, who struggled to communicate with humans. After all, he said, humans were fourth-dimensional light at one time before leaving the spirit world. Each of us is born with the innate ability to see spirits, but as we age, society and our parents interfere. They teach us to be ordinary and we, in turn, endeavor to remain that way. If we see ghosts or spirits, we tell ourselves it is simply our imagination.

In the spirit of open-mindedness, I halfheartedly participated in the group exercise and attempted to reach out to the willow that branched above me. "With humility, go back to your inner child—to your playful enchanted world," the leader said. Right away, herbalists around me saw spirits and heard voices. But I was a fourth-dimensional reject and just sat puzzled and quiet in the lotus position on the grass. I never really had a playful childhood, because at nine years of age, I washed dishes, cleaned, and cooked. I had no time for fairies or imaginary friends, and now I didn't really believe they existed.

Another herbal teacher, Adrienne Roan Bear, also gave me advice. "Go when the morning dew is freshest and the plants are most active." She added, "Rue is the spiritual protector and she should guide you."

I took a small sprig of my rue, whom I have come to know because I planted her near the door of my clinic. Rue's small delicate leaves reach up sensitively to the sky. At first glance, it is only her delicate personality she shows to the world, but on a deeper level, rue can be toxic when consumed. Having been used for generations for herbal-induced abortions, rue has many spiritual ties. She is an herb that recognizes both human darkness and light.

Cool morning fog enveloped the garden and rue and me. I hovered among my familiar plants and waited for a sign—a wiggle of a leaf or a hushed voice—but nothing happened. My left brain kept interfering, and I worried that the neighbors might wonder why I was talking to myself all alone in the garden. It was no good. I remembered, after trying all day in the workshop, dusting myself off and saying, "No one in her right mind would sit and talk to plant spirits."

Sitting at my desk, in front of a huge pile of herbal medicine books, I read with Angel in mind. After many hours, I found no new treatment—no novel herbal mechanism or new active ingredients. Everything I found was something I had used before. I stared out at the plants in my backyard garden. What unwritten legends could they reveal? All the folklore throughout generations of Native peoples and ancestral medicine was right there in my own backyard. It was not knowledge I longed for, but intuition, not textbook intellect, but healing that would come only from my own receptivity.

Time was running out; Angel was getting sicker, and so I finally returned to the safety of my desk and textbooks. My green lamp was turned up but still the room was in shadow. I read about active ingredients and enzymatic reactions and chemistry and, just as in college chemistry, I fell asleep, only this time with my face planted on top of *The Yoga of Herbs.* I had been in the middle of reading a scientific explanation of how woolly mullein helps soothe and restore damaged mucosal linings, like those of the lungs, intestines, and bladder. If someone had told me what would happen next, I certainly would not have believed them.

I wasn't sure if I was awake or sleepwalking. With a rush of birdsong, at five in the morning I went out to the garden as if I had been called there. Wind grappled with my hair. I was unnerved by the wind's power and the plants' beckoning. A robin came to me and I felt more at peace hearing her familiar song. My neck was stiff from sleeping all night on my books, but I was surprised by how clearheaded I felt. Suddenly the tall woolly mullein I usually ignored in the back of my garden waved all her yellow flower stalks at me as if they were waving hands of ancient Shiva. Mullein called to me in the blue hue of the morning with one flower-spoke hand waving in front of the other. I approached her as she beckoned, stepping deeper into my garden to pick one of her leaves.

Now more birds were singing and chirping very loudly; it was as if there were a full orchestra present. I looked up to see a red-tailed hawk circling, smelling, watching. I could see everything from his vantage point, and I heard my grandfather's voice closer and clearer than ever before: "Open yourself, notice every leaf, every bird, use every sense, like we did on our walks." I wanted him to help me; Grampa was so wise about plants. As I flew high above my garden, I noticed more birds joining us, singing. I realized that I was not alone—I had so many helpers. For one suspended moment, we playfully dipped, dived, and flipped about effortlessly.

Like generations of doctors before me, I imagined what Angel's body was doing from the inside. Only now, with the blue morning light and a vast array of bird guides, I did more than imagine. In one moment, I'd taken flight, while in the very next I became small, then tiny, and finally microscopic. I entered Angel's weak body to fully explore it. I became smaller than a microscopic cell, smaller than a molecule, than the smallest piece of energy, and I moved as fast as light. I became a piece of life's energy force—the Qi that separates the living from the dead. Through shrinking, I could explore. Through exploration, I could understand.

Even though I was burrowed deep, zooming around inside Angel's body, I heard the plants speak for the first time. "Take me, Take me," slippery coltsfoot whispered, low to the ground. My scientific mind knew she would be a great mucilaginous soother for Angel's dry, weakened air sacs. "No, not that leaf; I need that one. Here, take this one." I took a few of her leaves from the bottom. With mullein and coltsfoot in hand, I flew faster than a bird or any known entity. There were thousands of bursts of color and light surrounding me. Finally, I arrived at Angel's place of essence storage—a fading, flickering blue light between her kidneys. I used my leaves to strengthen the fire. Like an internal smudging, the smoking leaves cleaned and strengthened her kidneys just as the sweetgrass or sage that Native healers burn rids a place of bad spirits.

The thickened, spiculated leaves of lungwort rustled impatiently at my feet, calling me without words. Her white circular patches resembled the part of the lung she helped: alveoli or air sacs; and the tiny hairlike protrusions that covered her were similar to the microscopic villi of the lung. At once I knew my next stop would be the giant, cavernous air sacs, like caves along Angel's backbone. There were white strands of cobweb-like scar tissue hanging from the walls, shrinking air capacity after many months of illness. I sprinkled lungwort tea at the base of each cobweb and cleaned the sacs. I flittered hastily and soon Jing, or essence, followed me into each unexplored corner. Kidney essence needed help; alone, it was not strong enough to break down scar tissue.

I heard hearty comfrey loudly; she was a plant that took over conversations as well as gardens. "Hey, Donna, here!" I picked her strong, thick, almost prickly leaves. She would provide strength for Angel's weak body, for there is perhaps not a tougher, heartier plant. With comfrey, I went to Angel's paper-thin crop. It was supposed to grind up food and move it through, but instead it sat there. Comfrey was so strong. She could toughen the crop lining and heal the stretched-out walls.

I left Angel's body and grew big and slow again. I couldn't believe what had just happened in my own garden! I didn't know if the plants would ever engage me again like that, but for now, I was thrilled to have finally made contact with such powerful allies. Part of me was thrilled, and the other part was trying to remember if I had drunk too much wine the night before. Was it possible to actually hear plants talking?

My chosen fresh herbs were too cold and lacked energy. I needed help warming the Kidney, the Spleen, and the Lung. I wanted warming, fluid-supporting, nourishing herbs, so I added dried astragalus, cat's claw, pau d' arco, and cardamom from the amber bottles on my shelves. These herbs warm and strengthen the immune system. I brewed the concoction on my stove, and Chris began giving Angel the formula that day. Between the new herbal tea and a few more acupuncture visits, Angel regained and maintained a normal white blood cell count. She began to eat again.

Sometimes in the first light of the morning, my garden still takes on otherworldly airs. Every time I see my ten-foot mullein flailing her flower spikes in the wind, I wonder if she is trying to tell me something. When Angel gently takes hold of my finger during treatments, I think about the generations of animals and people healed by doctors who follow their guided instinctive intuition. In the process of treating Angel, I learned to listen to our vast and powerful plant allies in a new way.

Your Pet's Immune System

The immune system is vital for life; we are still learning more about it every day. If it is strong, the body can fight almost any infection. With weakness comes the opportunity for viruses and bacteria to grow in numbers and cause illness. The immune system consists of three major interrelated and interdependent subsystems. The first one is the B-lymphocyte cell system, which conveys humoral immunity and is programmed to create antibodies. When we do an antibody titer, we are looking for products of the B-cell line—namely, specific antibodies.

The second part of the immune system is the T-lymphocyte cell line, which conveys cell-mediated immunity, or CMI. It is the system that becomes affected in human AIDS and the similar feline retrovirus disease FIV. Both B- and T-lymphocyte cell immunity have lifetime or so-called immune memory from past encounters with infectious or other antigens. They are like armies that could easily conquer past enemies.

The third arm of the immune system is nonspecific immunity, in which giant macrophages and white blood cells go around like big Pac-Men gobbling up bacteria, viruses, and other foreign agents or proteins. We can measure antibody levels, T-cell numbers, and white blood cells with blood tests. Thus, we can tell how the immune system is doing quantitatively but not qualitatively—it is tough to measure how these cells are performing.

While Western medicine is good at suppressing the immune system by using steroids and chemotherapeutic agents, it is not as good at safely strengthening or balancing it. With regard to raising low white blood cell counts, holistic medicine really shines. Acupuncture can boost white blood cell counts and B-cells, can elevate natural killer-cell activity, and can stimulate the production of red blood cells.

When treating a weak immune system with herbs, we must consider the specific energetics of the patient. Energetically, it gets quite complicated because some infections are considered hot while others are cold and are caused by long-term debilitation. For example, if a cat has a low white blood cell count, and she is aged, has weak pulses, and has a pale tongue, an herbalist would want to use herbs that not only strengthen her immune system but also warm her on a very deep level. If a young dog has kennel cough, a relatively hot condition, pants a lot, likes to lie on concrete instead of carpets, and drinks lots of water, herbalists would use herbs that boost the immune system but also cool and detoxify the body.

Whether a patient's body is cold or hot can be difficult to assess, especially because in Chinese medical thought there are common inflammatory conditions that arise from "false heat" or a deep internal Qi deficiency (cold condition). Experienced holistic practitioners and herbalists can diagnose the difference and choose herbs, homeopathic medicines, or acupuncture points that strengthen the immune system to aid in fighting infection.

One of the most frustrating things about interacting with veterinarians practicing Western medicine is the degree to which they want to blame inflammation on infection. Just because there is heat in the body does not mean there are causative agents. Many bacteria are considered normal flora. Like Yin and Yang, there is a balance between Eastern and Western medical thought. Antibiotics do save lives, especially for bodies whose immune systems have become weak. Take your pet to the veterinarian, but try the safe super-duper immune-boosting herbal tea on the following page to supplement conventional medication.

The most important question to ask before using herbal teas is: What part of my pet's body is the weakest? Different herbs act on different locations. For example, if your pet has chronic or recurrent respiratory infections, the treatment might be different than if your pet has recurrent skin or bladder infections.

You can tell that your pet has an imbalanced immune system if his white blood cell count is repeatedly low or his globulins are chronically high; the veterinarian finds enlarged lymph nodes that are noncancerous; and he gets sick often. You can buy any of the herbs listed in these recipes at any shop that sells dried herbs in bulk. The three teas are all prepared in the same way, and directions are given at the end, on page 174.

General Immune-Booster Herbal Tea

Good for chronic or recurrent infections. Use in conjunction with your veterinarian's advice or just to keep your pet healthy. All herbs are in their raw, whole form.

1½ quarts low-sodium chicken broth or water
1 approximately 2-by-8-inch piece astragalus root (warming)
¼ cup cut rose hips (warming)
¼ cup cut pau d'arco bark (cooling)
¼ cup cut alfalfa leaf (nutritive; cooling)
¼ cup cut gotu kola leaves (cooling; cleans and feeds the immune system; adrenal support)
¼ cup cut cat's claw bark (neutral)
2 tablespoons chlorella powder

Respiratory-Support Herbal Tea

To aid with the healing of kennel cough, pneumonia, infectious bronchitis, and sinusitis. This tea can be given along with the General Immune-Booster Herbal Tea above.

1½ quarts low-sodium chicken broth or water
⅓ cup cut echinacea leaves (cooling)
¼ cup cut Oregon grape or goldenseal root or 2 tablespoons powdered herb
¼ cup cut marshmallow root (demulcent; slightly cooling)
¼ cup cut mullein leaves (demulcent; cooling)
⅛ cup grated fresh gingerroot (warming)
⅛ cup cut elecampane root (warming)

Urinary Support Herbal Tea

For cats with sterile cystitis, chronic or recurrent bladder infections, or, in Chinese medicine, Damp Heat invading the urinary bladder. This tea works best without the addition of other herbal teas.

    1½ quarts low-sodium chicken broth or water
    ⅓ cup cut yarrow flowers (cooling; clears blood in urine)
    ¼ cup cut Oregon grape or goldenseal root or 2 tablespoons
      powdered herb
    ¼ cup cut plantain leaves (cooling; astringent—dries mucus)
    ¼ cup *Uva ursi* leaves (cooling; cleans bladder wall)
    ¼ cup cut corn silk or marshmallow root (cooling; demulcent—soothing)

Combine all of the ingredients in a large stainless steel or ceramic saucepan, cover, and simmer over low heat for 20 minutes. Remove from the heat and set the covered pan in a cool place for 6 to 10 hours. Strain the tea, and discard the solids.

Keeping: The General Immune-Booster Herbal Tea will last for 10 days in the refrigerator, while the Respiratory and Urinary teas will last 3 weeks because of the addition of the antimicrobial, berberine-containing herbs goldenseal or Oregon grape root. I recommend freezing half of the tea in ice cube trays, and thawing as needed for later use. Store the ice cubes for up to one year, in a freezer bag to avoid freezer burn. One ice cube will last for a few days. Bring to room temperature before using.

Dosing: Give 1 tablespoon of tea per 25 pounds of the pet's weight for 10 to 14 days, although it is safe to use for extended periods—even months. The average cat weighs 10 pounds, so a dose would be about ½ tablespoon twice daily. It can be given either by syringe or with a small amount of food. For birds and other exotic pets, the dose is 1 milliliter per kilogram, so the average cockatoo gets 0.5 cc twice a day, on a cracker.

THESE TEAS ARE NOT MEANT TO REPLACE VETERINARY CARE but, rather, to augment it. (See Resources, page 263.)

HEALING CHARLIE HORSE

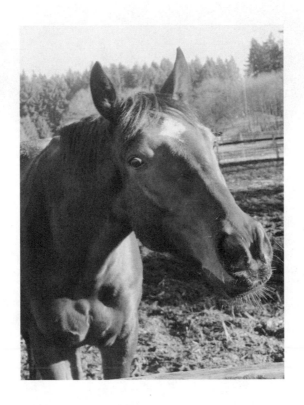

My thoughts are clearest when I ride Charlie, my six-year-old thoroughbred. He has taught me a lot since I adopted him on a rainy Monday in November 1998. I have used chiropractic, acupuncture, herbs, and homeopathy to fix his back, reduce his swellings, and heal his cuts and contusions. Today my big bay gelding is healthy. As he quickens the pace toward home, I notice the gleam of his coat in the setting sun; his long walking stride is like a powerful undercurrent beneath me. We are alone, he and I, which I know to be dangerous. I could fall; Charlie could get loose or injure himself. But we have built three years of trust in each other and the trail gives us a sense of meditative peace.

We are far from other people, surrounded by thick Pacific Northwest cedar, spruce, and hemlock trees, and dense, lush, green bracken fern. The air is invigorating, like a freshly cut Christmas tree. Birds drift and dart to and fro, chirping in rhythm to our footfalls, which echo through the ravine. There is bright green moss in every possible space, hanging from hemlock and cedar trees and covering old stumps. Sun rays glide down through the forest canopy like a multitude of spotlights on the natural beauty surrounding us. Charlie drops his head and sighs.

Although my equine companion is only six years old, he has been retired from the racetrack for three years. Horses often live into their thirties, so age three is early for retirement. In fact, at the age of six, he now has all his adult teeth and his bones have just fully matured. His body is a conglomeration of tendons, ligaments, joints, and bones working perfectly together to allow me to ride. In order to remain free from lameness, his teeth must be even, with no sharp edges; his joints must be free from inflammation; and his tendons must glide past one another with the smoothness of silk and the strength of rope. There must be perfect timing of all parts to allow his half-ton body to move with ease.

As a child, I didn't know about equine anatomy, or the reality of the racetrack, but I loved it. I glorified the racetrack because, like my grandmother's humming in the morning, watching horse races brought my tattered family closer. Grandma would make popcorn and my job was mixing lemonade. My grandmother, mother, brother, and I watched, in awe of the sleek thoroughbreds, the Kentucky Derby, the Preakness, and the Belmont. I can remember the thrill of the announcer's voice, the scream of the crowd, and the thunder of beautiful horses running with all their hearts. Gathered around our small color television in a cozy, humid apartment outside Boston, my family would munch on popcorn, feeling envious of the jockeys. How exciting it would be to ride one of the fastest animals in the world—weightlessly, effortlessly gliding, as if your body was one with the horse. As they galloped down the homestretch, we jumped to our feet, fists flailing at the sky.

Finally, after I spent years cleaning stalls to work off the cost of riding lessons, my mother bought me my first pony, Lady. The excitement of having my first horse was captured in an enlarged photograph my grandparents took. There I was, thirteen years old, short brown hair blowing in the cool fall wind. I sat astride my dappled Appaloosa. Her mane rippled in the gusty breeze. A thread of spunk shot through her old bones and in the picture, she jogged in place—two feet off the ground. My smile, shaky with teenage self-doubt, nevertheless revealed my happiness on that hilltop with the sun setting behind us.

Lady was no racehorse, but I pretended she was. She would turn and look at me suspiciously: a crazy girl shortening her stirrups to jockey length and sitting up in half seat—the jockey position. Little by little, Lady and I ran faster around the outdoor arena crowded with show jumps. My eyes teared, my hair swished back from under my hard hat. At my imaginary warp speed, stationary objects blurred. I practiced balancing with my seat off the saddle as if I were the most famous woman jockey in the world.

Years later, while attending clinical rotations in vet school, each student cared for many broken-down horses. We spent many hours, day after day, walking up and down the huge corridors in the large-animal teaching hospital at WSU in Pullman, Washington. The smell of cedar shavings, timothy hay, and Betadine antiseptic cleaner wafted through the air. We bandaged injured racehorses, wrapped their bowed tendons, flushed their wounds, and hosed their inflamed joints. We performed bone scans on their tired bodies and helped surgeons remove bone chips from the darkest crevasses of their joints.

Charlie is not the glamorous racehorse I dreamed of riding when I was a child; instead, he is a broken survivor of the racetrack. Scars on his legs tell the untold story of the reality of the Sport of Kings. But Charlie is lucky compared to some.

Lucy's Life on the Track

Through the years, my experience with the racetrack was largely as an observer. I spent time at breeding and training barns. I tagged along with trainers and horse friends, and later, I occasionally followed some equine vet friends while they worked. I did admire the hard workers on the track. The backstretch life is not easy. If their horses do not win, many of the jockeys and trainers don't get paid.

I remember witnessing my first horse birthing, at a thoroughbred breeding farm. At the center of acres of grassy pastures was a barn consisting of shed rows. Each shed row housed about thirty mares in separate box stalls divided by metal gates. Through rusty metal bars, a foal eagerly swished onto the straw. When her spindly front legs poked through the milky amniotic sac, she stood up, shaking, and I saw the steam of her first exhale in the chill of the winter air. Her dam licked the foal's face and body clean. With one dim lightbulb shared between stalls, it was easy to see the bright white star on the foal's forehead and three glow-in-the-dark white socks.

The foal seemed filled with excitement at new things—raindrops on her back, the taste of salt licks, and the feeling of grass under her tiny hooves. The people who cared for her were amazed by the way Lucy boldly and fearlessly wandered away from her dam to places other foals did not go alone. Lucy investigated fallen branches from trees and the fences that surrounded her. Little by little she roamed farther from her mother, to the farthest reaches of the field.

One night she squeezed under the metal gate and playfully explored a dark aisle. Jorge, the barn manager, left early for his trailer that night so no one heard Lucy's dam whinnying for her filly. I imagined that Lucy could hear only her own small hooves and could see only the trees blowing vigorously at the other end of the aisle. From the evidence found in the morning, she had strewn a box of stale doughnuts all over the aisleway before returning to her distraught mother. Jorge and the others found Lucy standing outside her mother's stall the next morning. Since no harm had come to her, she was named "Lucky Lucy."

My friend sold Lucy to a racetrack trainer named Al. He had other reasons to call her Lucky—Lucy was fast, and I mean real fast. When she was a year old, she sold for $30,000. I heard the sale pavilion announcer rattle off, "Hip eighty-one sold to the man in tweed for thirty." That day, Lucy was named after the number (81) taped to both hips, but later, when she would arrive at the track, she would be known by the number of her tattoo, visible under every racehorse's lip.

I helped my racetrack veterinarian friend, Teresa, on one sale day. I followed Teresa down the aisle carrying some blank forms, a clipboard, and an endoscope. I put Lucy's halter on and slipped a chain under her top lip. Lucky Lucy flared her nostrils and snorted a little at our unwelcome presence. Her eyes bulged with terror. Her body was not her own; every inch of it was probed and studied, even though what makes a winner often cannot be quantified or even understood. Some horses can overcome their anatomical defects with spirit, heart, and drive that can carry them on crooked legs first over the finish line.

Teresa passed the long hose into Lucy's nose. I breathed softly, telling her it would soon be over. If Lucy's airways were narrowed or her laryngeal cartilages didn't close entirely, her life as a racehorse might never materialize. I was secretly hoping Teresa would find a problem so that Lucy would be deemed unfit for racing, but Teresa wrote on the record "no abnormalities found."

We were turning to leave Lucy's stall when a man met us in the doorway. He held a brown sale book and had his finger pressing a page inside; I guessed it was the page with Lucy's bloodline and statistics. "You the vet?" he asked in a gruff voice, without the distinguished air his flat English cap suggested. Teresa was hurriedly trying to get the rest of the horses scoped, but money talked on sale day.

"I am," she answered, packing the endoscope into its box. He was wearing a tweed coat that didn't button over his belly, and rolls of tanned skin hung over a thick gold chain around his neck.

"You think she's a winner?" He ignored me, turning to face the horse.

"Just know she's got good airways," Teresa said, leaving him to shut the door.

180

"I get sick of all these trainers sometimes. I know they are really running the show," she said as we both walked fast to the next barn.

"Do you ever feel as if you are a puppet? Do you ever feel bad about what happens to the horses?" I asked.

"Sure, sometimes, especially when I first started, but now I like some of the trainers and don't think they push the horses too hard. I try not to think about it." Her answer left me feeling unsatisfied. Teresa and I became close in vet school because we worked in clinics together. I had always wanted to be tough like her, but now, as I looked into her eyes, I realized that she could not hold up her veterinary oath and also be a racetrack vet. Her first priority was not to the horses but to the trainers and owners.

Teresa's career was in sharp contrast to what I thought veterinary life was like. When I was eighteen, my second horse, Bill, pulled his back out after I jumped a tight course. The poor big chestnut gelding could barely walk so I called Floyd, an old-time healer from the Longacres backstretch. He was a tall, kind African-American man with sunken cheeks and a loose laugh. I trusted him with Bill immediately because anyone could tell that if there was one thing Floyd knew, despite having no formal education, it was horses. He had worked on the backstretch since he was fifteen and learned about horses from his father, who also worked on the racetrack.

Although Floyd would not reveal his secret muscle-relaxing remedy, I saw him pour DMSO (a strong solvent that penetrates fast into the bloodstream to carry other herbs or medications into the back's sore muscles), some herbal glycerin concoction, and liniment into a bowl and stir it up. I stood in the stable doorway in awe of this backstretch healer standing on top of a loosened hay bale. After gloving his hands to protect them from the DMSO, he rubbed the concoction into Bill's painful back.

"Got two heavy winter rugs?" he asked me, his eyes still focused on his patient.

I was so worried about Bill I thought I would cry. "But it's summer and real hot lately," I questioned him.

"What we need here is a good ol' sweatin," he answered in a quiet monotone that conveyed his command of horsemanship. I didn't question another word and retrieved the heaviest blankets from the bottom of my tack trunk. Floyd gave my horse some homeopathic pellets and some muscle relaxers. The next day, Bill was caked with dried sweat but he was as good as new. I thought about how different Teresa was from Floyd, even though they had both worked on the track.

I saw Lucy months later, on the last night she would race. She weaved from side to side at the front of her stall and ignored her full hay net. She was becoming "stall crazy." The horses on either side of her munched quietly on their hay and rested in the back of their box stalls.

"Well, I think you should give her more bute," her trainer said, believing that the anti-inflammatory injection would get her through this last race of the season. Judging from his surefooted stance, crossed arms, and baseball hat tipped up, I was pretty sure he had made up his mind.

"Did you try wrapping her legs at night or putting clay poultices on her knees?" Teresa asked. She was uncomfortable about giving Lucy another injection, because only a certain amount of bute was allowed by state regulations; also, because it strongly masks pain, Lucy might injure herself further.

"Yeah, we did it all, Doc; she's still sore," Lucy's trainer assured Teresa. Teresa sighed and then gave all the injections. She injected some yellow solution into Lucy's jugular vein, which was scarred from previous injections. She said it was Lasix, given to prevent racehorses from bleeding into their lungs. Most horses at the track are given this drug because they are exerted beyond their physiological capability. Bleeding can occur when the pulmonary vessels leak blood during the exertion of racing. This can lead to pleuritis, pneumonia, and even death. Sometimes jockeys also take Lasix because it dehydrates the body, so they can weigh in under the limit. Teresa gave a second injection, a small amount of clear phenylbutazone, or bute.

As is protocol before racing, four hours before the race her water buckets were removed and ice boots were placed on Lucy's legs. She was groomed and shiny; every stray piece of mane was combed or removed because, as well as speed, image mattered tonight. The public would see only a beautiful chestnut filly. But as I looked at Lucy, I worried. Her immature bones, the drugs, and her emotional stress left me feeling uneasy.

That night I saw my first and last live horse race. I sat next to Jorge in the grandstands and Lucy's trainer sat behind us. He was sucking down a Miller and had a bedraggled cigar hanging from one corner of his mouth. To our left, we could see Lucy and the other horses parading counterclockwise, without saddles, for public inspection. Above the activity, the moon held still in the sky but was barely visible past the huge lights of the statistics board. I saw a couple of jockeys pacing and smoking, anxiously waiting to mount. I wasn't sure if it was the weigh-in or the race making them nervous.

"The purse is five thousand dollars, so Lucy is running against some of the faster horses," Jorge said and then fell silent. Although I worried about Lucy, I settled into the crowd and their excitement rubbed off on me a bit. For a moment, as the crowd grew anxious around me, I remembered the enthusiasm of my youth. I imagined my family together again and how grand we would have felt seeing a real live race! But when I saw Lucy trotting sideways toward the start gate, my stomach tightened with worry. The other horses were already lined up. *Ding ding ding.* The bell rang and in half a blink, the announcer screamed, "They're off!"

Behind me, I could see Lucy's trainer lean forward and mutter to himself. As the horses ran, their sleek bodies moved like the elegant ripple of a ballroom full of nineteenth-century satin gowns. Hooves pounded, dirt flew, and the slap of jockeys' whips at every stride struck me like an electric cattle prod. The spectators, including Al, rushed to the white gate along the homestretch. I winced when Lucy rounded the homestretch— the pointed toe grabs on her forefeet slipped to the outside. In front of the large, lit statistics board, the horses pounded themselves faster, and I felt the jar in my own joints as the horses crossed the finish line. Lucy was in front, over the wire by a few lengths.

I stopped, breathless. Lucy was unable to walk. Her jockey swung his small body off and within an instant there was a small crowd around her. Teresa and some other vets drove a horse ambulance next to Lucy. I stood frozen. Her trainer was already by her side and I saw him tip his head back, upset, frustrated, powerless, while Lucy's front leg hung weightlessly in an unnatural twist below the knee. I felt my heart pound.

As if freed from the starting gate, I imagined that I ran fast, as if I were on the drugs, down past the murmuring crowd, past the gatekeepers, just to see Lucy being driven away, to be hidden, concealed like a prisoner about to be destroyed. There was commotion, arguing and angry words. I imagined that I could reach out to help her, but in the end, only my outstretched fingers grazed her, as if touching a ghostly shadow. In her last minutes, she would feel a familiar needle, but this time one on each side of her neck, sinking into both jugulars at the same time. Her young body would fall uncontrollably to the ground, and the world she had tried so hard to run away from would suddenly go black.

I shudder now when I think Charlie might have suffered as Lucy did. I wonder what would have happened to this extrovert whose big brown eyes exude kindness. Everywhere Charlie goes, horses line their fences to

183

greet him and people reach out to pet him. Many people believe it was his personality that saved him.

Charlie's Second Career

Instead of pushing Charlie as hard as some horses, his trainer used the two-year-old as his coffee horse. Socializing came easy to both horse and trainer, and together, they would visit anyone in the backstretch shed rows who could chat. Rumor has it (and rumors spread fast on the track) that after a few weeks, the coffee chat list grew longer. Soon, everyone on the backstretch knew Charlie the horse and looked for his comical curlicue star. After a few months, the horse had a fan club of horse groupies, mostly mares, that neighed for a visit. Even now, when I lead Charlie to his pasture, I feel as if I am walking with a popular politician! Both mares and geldings pause to rub noses with him.

But life on the track was not usually much fun for the big bay gelding. He was ink branded, just like Lucy, under his lip with a bright blue "K22036." Charlie won his first race at the track, giving false hope to his trainer, owner, and jockey. Geldings have twice the breakdown rate of females because, owing to their inability to breed, they are considered more disposable so they are pushed harder. Charlie had eight starts as a two-year-old. If horses are raced too hard, each small injury accumulates, growing more severe, like an avalanche as it falls down a mountainside. Eventually, Charlie needed two surgeries to remove bone chips in his knee. Because Charlie's trainer opted not to continue pushing his gossip buddy, he retired Charlie, turning him onto pasture to rest for several months.

In 1998, Teresa called to see if I wanted to take Charlie. It was a tough decision. Because my holistic practice had slowed down for the holidays, I was still working all-night emergency shifts to make ends meet. Taking on another five-hundred-dollar-a-month expense did not seem feasible. I spent the next month deciding whether to take Charlie.

My mother and grandmother were both morning decision makers. If they had a decision to make, big or small, it was always made before seven, as if it had had to brew overnight. I remember my grandmother scuffling into my room several days after Grampa died. She told me that she had decided the flowers from his funeral should not be wasted. "We'll make small bouquets for all the guests to take home. Paul would like that."

Years before, my mother had exclaimed at six in the morning, "We are moving to Seattle—well, Tacoma, actually." We had never heard of Seattle, but she had been offered a job at a four-year university. What could my brother or I say? We were still half asleep.

Following this long line of early decision makers, I decided at seven A.M. to take Charlie. I missed having a horse in my life, and he really needed acupuncture and chiropractic on a regular basis. In vet school, I had begun to learn what racing does to horses. Adopting Charlie brought the painful truth home. For the first few weeks, he pointed, or stuck his injured leg in front of him at night. I comforted him during his uncomfortable episodes. I led him around the neighborhood. He ate grass and became acquainted with all the local horses who ran up to the gate to meet him.

Rehabilitating him was a step-by-step process over the course of several months. I rummaged through an old tack box and pulled out a tool called a hoof tester. It looks like a big aluminum clamp with a Pac-Man-like mouth. I opened this tool and clamped it onto Charlie's right front foot. This instrument is supposed to put pressure on precise locations and test for pain. I squeezed down across the coffin bone, the lowest bone under the hoof, and diagonally over the navicular bone, a small, wafer-shaped bone in the back of the hoof. I also pushed across the bulbs of the heel. *No pain. Good.* I repeated this hoof test on all his feet. Although Charlie did not have particularly strong, large hooves, he didn't have any additional problems in the joints of his feet. Not knowing the way his new owner would push and poke at him, he stared at me in wonder while I checked him out.

Thoroughbreds are not bred for good hooves, and Charlie is no exception. His are small and crumbly. There is an old expression, "No feet, no horse," and I thought about ways to improve his feet. I gave him supplements to increase the biotin and methionine in his diet and I asked my farrier to shorten Charlie's toes. At the track, toes are left long to get an edge over the other racehorses but, unfortunately, this practice puts more force on the tendons. Eventually, a form of farriery called "natural balance" helped Charlie's feet the most.

Charlie's tendons were not bowed but chronically inflamed, so I bandaged his legs for support the first month. His knee swelled once after he got rambunctious and scraped up against a fence, so I applied herbal comfrey poultices and hosed his leg daily to treat the swollen laceration. I did acupuncture to relieve the pain. After a few weeks, he improved, but he still did not appreciate a saddle on his sore back.

185

If there was a weakness in my conventional equine veterinary training, it was backs and teeth. We seemed to learn next to nothing about how to diagnose, palpate, or treat equine dental or spinal problems. In veterinary school, I remember memorizing lists of anatomical names, the importance of which was never discussed and the application to a real live animal never mentioned. We learned the contents of the intervertebral foramen (the space between each vertebra); specifically, the arteries, veins, nerves, and lymphatics located there, but not until animal chiropractic school did I learn the importance of these structures. Chiropractic misalignments can pinch blood vessels and impair the flow of lymph, disrupting the immune system.

Charlie and I stood facing each other in a dimly lit aisleway one month after I got him. His legs were no longer a problem, but every time I tried to put the saddle on him, he threw his head up and hollowed his back, arching it away from touch or pressure. Being the laid-back fellow that he is, he held no grudges. I slid my chiropractic bale (a large, solid but light-weight hay-bale-shaped stepping stool) along his right side and climbed on top of it, laying my hands on his back to examine him. I started from the tail end, on his sacrum, and worked forward. I carefully felt whether it was centered or skewed, whether the base had popped up slightly, and whether it was painful. Gently, I rocked it from side to side and Charlie swished his tail and flipped his head, his form of complaint. I adjusted the sacrum by bracing against the large triangular bone and thrusting slightly. He allowed me to work my way up his spine and was practically asleep at the end of the treatment.

Acupuncture would be a constant treatment for Charlie for years to come. Every few months, I slipped needles into points to restore full function to a neighboring joint, to help with swelling or pain along a meridian, and to help him heal. Like most horses, he did not seem to even notice the needles, because compared to the joint and back pain he was experiencing, small acupuncture needles might have felt no worse than a tiny, biting fly. After a few minutes with the needles in place, his lower lip would start to droop as if he were sedated. Inserting acupuncture needles causes the release of the horse's own endorphins. Over a few weeks, the treatments permanently eradicated his pain and muscle spasms. He did not mind the saddle and I started riding him, on trails and in the arena, and even began jumping him some—which he still loves.

Like the rest of him, Charlie's teeth were not too healthy. He began to shake his head a lot when the bit was in his mouth. Horses' teeth continually grow. On the open plains, coarse brush and grasses do a good job of grinding the wild horses' teeth evenly. Now, with soft hays and grain, horses' teeth need regular floating, or rasping, especially if the upper and lower jaws don't meet evenly. The angle of the teeth and the table, or where the upper and lower teeth meet, tell the age of the animal. "Don't look a gift horse in the mouth" refers to being able to tell a horse's age by its teeth.

In Charlie's case, he was young but had so many small pokey spikes and uneven spurs that it was a wonder he would tolerate a bit in his mouth at all. Feeling as though my training in floating teeth did not lend itself to sticking a large rasp in Charlie's mouth, I called another vet to do it. Unfortunately, the vet did not sedate Charlie before placing a speculum in the mouth and really doing the job right. In fact, she charged me seventy-five dollars to blindly run the blade a few times in his mouth.

I was greatly disgruntled and finally called a school for horse dentists in Idaho. Veterinarians can go to this school for additional training, but equine dental schools are not without controversy because nonveterinarians are also enrolled there. One of the head veterinarian instructors and his partner just happened to be working in the Seattle area and came out to help with Charlie.

They were Idaho cowboys, the two-stepping, big-belt-buckle kind, and they handled Charlie's mouth as carefully as if he were a pussycat. They sedated him and placed a large metal speculum in his mouth so he could not close it on our hands. A horse's cheek, or back, teeth extend back farther than most people realize, about a foot from the soft muzzle. Tooth problems can cause lameness, as horses attempt to move their whole body away from a painful edge. We used a flashlight to examine his teeth.

Charlie's teeth were uneven. There were steps and waves and spurs and spikes. In fact, to my chagrin, most of the abnormalities described in an equine dentist's manual existed in my horse's mouth. Given the degree of pathology, the veterinary dentists were forced to use power tools instead of gentle rasping, sending small pieces of teeth and saliva flying. Luckily my ex-racehorse was so tired from the sedation, his head hung to the ground. For five days, I let Charlie's mouth heal and did not ride him. Afterward, he went along as happily as could be, no head shaking, no ear pinning, and, above all, no pain.

Today, Charlie is a handsome big bay gelding. His three white socks and squiggly star gleam in the sunlight. When we come home from a trail ride, he stops, as he always does, square in front of the barn door, patiently awaiting my dismount. In his stall, Charlie and I wade in a bed of cedar shavings and timothy hay. I put his saddle and bridle away, and brush his dark brown coat. I lift each of his four hooves, and use my hoof pick to clean out rocks and dirt from the sole and from around each frog, or single toe. I give him his favorite post-trail-ride treat—a large red apple. He bites off half and slobbers white foam onto the floor.

I let him roll to scratch his back. He drops to the ground and rocks onto his back with all four legs in the air, and he scratches on the right and then on the left as if he is trying to make a sloppy snow angel. Afterward, for a minute, he stays down in the shavings, all four legs tucked underneath him, his head at knee level. Horses feel vulnerable while lying down to sleep, and by his doing so in my presence, I know that Charlie trusts me as if I were part of his herd. I sit down beside him, and hold his neck. Unconsciously, I run my hand down his jugular groove. There are no large scars from injections, no drugs coursing through his veins, and there is no pain from surgery. We rest there in the stall together, he and I. Charlie's life on the track has become only a memory—except for the tattoo and a few blemishes only I can see.

Racehorse Woes

There are hundreds of racehorses who die annually in the United States because of fatal breakdowns. Factors that contribute to racehorse breakdowns include: hardness of track footing, types of shoes, interval between races, amount of medication, frequency of races, and sex of horse. Geldings are generally pushed harder. Many people are confused as to why horses are normally euthanized after suffering fractures. There are many reasons for this, including the following.

HORSES ARE MEANT
TO STAND ON FOUR FEET

They don't lie down often and can even sleep standing up. When they are injured, they are afraid to lie down because it would be too hard to get back up. Standing on three legs over weeks can cause lameness.

BLOOD SUPPLY

There is little blood supply to the lower limbs of the horse because there is no muscle below the knee, or the hock. An artery or nerve is easily damaged because there is little tissue protecting these important structures. If a body is injured in one place, normally there is collateral circulation—other vessels will take over and compensate for the injury. The lower leg of the horse has few collateral options. The end result is that after just a few weeks, the foot below a fracture will become necrotic and infected.

THE ECONOMICS OF THE INDUSTRY

The cost of saving a horse with nursing care, bandages, cast changes, and antibiotics is in the tens of thousands, with no guarantee of recovery. The odds get worse for fractures above the knee and hocks because the bones are so large. Large bones mean blood supply is limited and therefore healing is slow.

A DISPOSABLE COMMODITY?

It might not be fatal breakdowns that are most troubling, but the way the industry treats racehorses as disposable. If horses started racing at an older age, their joints might be better preserved for subsequent careers. Many ex-racehorses end up in slaughterhouses. It is not just slow racehorses that have sad stories. Over his life, the racehorse Exceller won $1,654,003 by outstanding performances in France, England, and North America. On April 7, 1997, instead of dying a peaceful death out at pasture, he died in a slaughterhouse. On August 9, 1999, he was inducted into the National Museum of Racing's Hall of Fame in Saratoga, New York. The juxtaposition of honor and lack of respect for the well-being of horses is standard in the racing industry.

RESCUE AND REHABILITATION

In the United Kingdom, perhaps under pressure from animal rights groups, the British Horseracing Board has initiated official industry-financed rehabilitation and emergency-care funds. So far, this collective industry-driven effort remains to be seen in the States. In the United States, although some private-interest racetrack groups donate to numerous unrelated nonprofit rescue organizations, most donations come from the public.

I would love to see government regulations, with off-track enforcement, mandate the following changes: racehorses being allowed to begin their careers only after maturity; the banning of unsafe shoes; the giving of fewer medications; and the limiting of numbers of starts per season. The horseracing industry should not be self-regulated.

RESOURCES

The Exceller Fund Racehorse Adoption Program: www.excellerfund.org
Thoroughbred Retirement Foundation: www.trfinc.org
    TRF is a nonprofit organization that provides lifetime retirement for thoroughbreds. TRF-operated farms in Connecticut, Florida, Kentucky, Massachusetts, Michigan, New Hampshire, New Jersey, New York, Virginia, Vermont, and Wisconsin are located in state correctional facilities, where the horses' caretakers are adult prison inmates and juvenile offenders who derive both emotional and educational benefits from pioneering TRF vocational programs in horse care.

> HOOVED ANIMAL HUMANE SOCIETY
> P.O. Box 400
> Woodstock, IL 60098
> www.hahs.org

Use any search engine (such as www.about.com, www.google.com, or www.yahoo.com). Type "Racehorse Rescue" in the search box to get a list of numerous nonprofit organizations.

CAT ON A HUNGER STRIKE

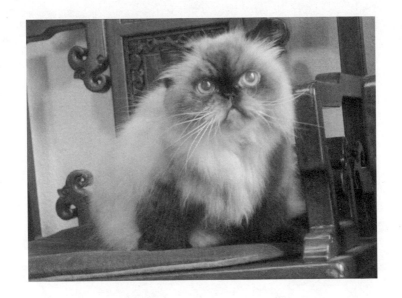

There was a quiet war brewing on the third floor of Seattle's Longview apartments, near the Globe Café where wonderful vegan cinnamon rolls bake every morning. It was every animal lover's nightmare: cat versus caretaker, neither side willing to give in to the other. The two parties had been squaring off on the tiled kitchen floor for two hours: Lana Hoolihan armed with cans and kibble on one side and Nikita, the squished-faced, fifteen-year-old seal point Himalayan on the other.

The stubborn beige cat sat in front of seven food bowls, front paws and bottom planted, tail flicking occasionally, immovable. His soft brown ears and tail made him resemble a cunning raccoon without the stripes. Armed with love and perseverance, Lana tried many tactics to get Nikita to eat.

First, the direct approach—Try It, You'll Like It—in which she plopped her forefinger in some cat food and then wiped it in Nikita's mouth. He backed away, stretching his head far from the food. That clearly had not gone well, so she attempted the Reverse Psychology method, in which she put the bowls away and pretended not to care if he ate. That also backfired; Nikita just disappeared back under the bed. At last, in quiet desperation, she tried the infamous I Want Some, So Should You tactic, pretending to eat Nikita's food. Nikita stared at Lana in disbelief as the spoon of tuna and chicken came closer and closer to her mouth. Afterward, she verbally faked her appreciation: "Yum, yum."

Nikita would not eat. And that was that. He had always been finicky, but this time he had gone to a new extreme. For several days, he walked by recently filled bowls as if they did not exist. His blue eyes peered at Lana from behind his flat face as if to say, "Hmph, you can't make me. So there." She tried every type of food on the market for cats: Friskies, Hill's,

Nutros; chicken, fish, liver, and beef. Then she extended the menu to the usual people food—deli turkey, canned tuna, canned sardines, pâté, consommé, and even cantaloupe. Not even a sniff of interest. And as if Lana weren't exhausted enough trying to help Nikita, her remaining energy was zapped by chronic fatigue syndrome—an illness that had plagued her for fifteen long years.

The battle between Nikita and Lana was born of mutual respect and compassion. There were many times, through the years of Lana's fatigue, when she might have given up, resigned to the degenerative path of her illness. With Lana lying exhausted on the couch, Nikita would sit nearby on the floor and make a guffawing sound. If Lana so much as raised an eyebrow at him, he chortled and started toward the bathroom. Lana couldn't help but follow. Loping past the kitchen water bowl, Nikita would look back at Lana to make sure she was following. Then he'd make a run for the bathroom, plant himself by the water bowl there, and look at Lana. Nikita waited with a gleam in his eye for Lana to pour the old water out and replace it with new water, even if she had just replaced it a few minutes before. Sniffing the fresh bowl of water, Nikita would twitch his whiskers the way Charlie Chaplin wiggled his mustache.

After the game reached its conclusion, Lana would head back to the couch with a lighter heart. Nikita would trot right behind her, and, as soon as she had settled herself back down, would begin cajoling her once again. One of the most frustrating aspects of her fatigue, Lana told me, was the way it affected her outward personality, adding weight to the levity with which she usually viewed the world. Lana saw that despite his hip and back problems, Nikita had chosen to adopt a playful attitude. And despite Lana's fatigue and her sluggish body, Nikita still recognized the merriment in her. He was worried about his beloved mistress; it was as if his care for her gave her cause to reevaluate her plight.

Now Lana was not going to give up on Nikita. After all, he had been finicky in the past. But of the two, Nikita is generally the stronger willed. His tactic is simple but clever: Wait it out and allow Lana's inevitable guilt to build. I saw Nikita's stubborn personality for myself when I went to visit him sometime later. When he wants to go out, he'll sit in front of the door and stare at the doorknob, sometimes for hours. Eventually, Lana will take him for a walk in the apartment courtyard with Koshka, his kitty roommate. When he has finished munching on grass or wandering around the garden, he climbs the stairs and sits staring at his caretaker. Koshka is usually not finished yet, but Nikita will wait and stare until he gets his way. I've rarely known such a determined creature.

During that fateful month of Nikita's vanishing appetite, Lana's chronic fatigue was worsening again. She regressed back to the point where all she could manage was work and caring for Nikita. Laundry went undone or sometimes unfolded, and, as luck would have it, Nikita would pee right on top of the pile. Sometimes she put a frozen dinner in the microwave but, by the time the bell went off, she lacked the strength to get up, take it out, and eat it. Since she would do anything for her cats, they often came before her health. Western medicine offered so little help for her illness that Lana doubted holistic medicine could improve her condition. She did start a yoga class, though, which helped.

About the same time that Lana and her cat went through his period of anorexia, I seemed to be going through a healing slump of my own. I sat in Seattle's gridlock traffic lamenting this to my own two dogs, Smudge and Sugar. Of the two, Sugar is the more patient with my ranting. A mid-size shepherd cross, Sugar is the only soul on earth who is truly interested in everything I say. I could see her wide empathetic eyes in my rearview mirror. "Why are some of my patients dying?" I asked her. "And why don't they build a damn train in this city?" Meanwhile, Smudge, my twenty-pound miniature black Lab mix and vet-school adoptee, sat by my side while I drove, as always. Smudge had been my copilot and best friend through at least five significant boyfriends over the past ten years. I had declared my profound love for each one to her over the years, and now, I think, she had sort of tuned me out. It's sad to be slighted by your own dog. In general, though, they are a great team, Smudge and Sugar, because Sugar listens and Smudge finds ways to direct me to answers.

I told Smudge and Sugar how I missed my grandmother Ruth, who had died the year before. She had always been my "giggle partner," and she seemed to have a knack for finding comedy in everything. Once she told me, "If you lose your sense of humor, life will only be black and white, drab, with no colors. And what is worse—the small details of life will over-whelm you. Then you will lose sight of your real purpose." When Grandma died, I lost my comical insight into life. Grandma could turn almost any situation into a "character-building event," and could see instantly that what sends some people into fits of anger or tears is actually trite in comparison with the importance of people's feelings. The only thing that really mattered to my grandmother was treating all beings with kindness and understanding. For that reason, animals flocked to her. As if they found solace in her levity, my own dogs would stick to her side when we were together. Maybe losing my comical view of the world was also negatively affecting my ability to help animals.

It was a grim time emotionally for me and physically for Nikita that month. For years, Nikita had battled back and hip arthritis, but now blood tests revealed Lana's worst fear: kidney disease. In Chinese medicine, weakness of the hind limbs and arthritis are often attributed to Kidney imbalances, but now those small problems had escalated.

The blood tests showed Nikita's blood urea nitrogen (BUN) to be five times the normal level and his creatinine at a threefold elevation. These are waste products that are excreted through the kidneys, if they are working. If the kidneys aren't functioning well, these normal waste products build up in the blood, causing toxic effects on the tissues, such as ulcers on the gums. In a desperate attempt to force more blood to the kidneys to detoxify faster, blood pressure increases. Urine tests showed that Nikita's kidneys weren't doing their job of reabsorbing water back into the body; instead they let much-needed water and electrolytes escape into the urine.

The vet told Lana that this deterioration was to be expected; after all, Nikita was fifteen years old and his kidneys were most likely failing. Through four separate visits to her conventional vet, Lana discovered that Nikita's failing kidneys were leaving him dehydrated, with a low potassium level. This dehydration occurs when microscopic renal tubules called nephrons become so dysfunctional they can't do their job of reabsorbing water or salts back into the body. Cats with kidney disease drink a lot and pee a lot because they are trying to maintain hydration.

Nikita also developed eye problems, common in these flat-faced, bulging-eyed cats. First he suffered a corneal ulcer, and then the veterinary ophthalmologist found inflammation around Nikita's optic nerve, visible only through careful examination of the back of his eyes. He was convinced the inflammation might be due to cancer.

Lana fretted about Nikita. Unfortunately, she was no stranger to losing cats. Her feline companion Sasha had been diagnosed with kidney disease and had died at only six years of age. Nikita's best feline friend and brother, Kahlua, died after he ate the ribbon off a package. The two brothers had been inseparable and spent most days sleeping intertwined, chest to chest, white whiskers pressed against black ones.

The depression Nikita now suffered reminded Lana of the time just after his feline brother died. Nikita had hidden under a wooden chair and refused to eat. Lana would lie on the floor and sing sideways, cheek against the hard wood, for however long it took to coax the sulking feline out into the open. It didn't surprise me when she described his health problems as originating from this grief. He began walking oddly at that time, and, Lana said, "His spine had a horrible sharp kink just behind the shoulders."

According to Lana, it was then that Nikita developed his aversion to litter boxes. Perhaps climbing in and out caused back pain. He had maintained this unexplained abhorrence ever since, peeing mainly on small bath rugs Lana kept piled for just this reason. If she forgot and left a pile of laundry or work papers in the living room, she would find Nikita's gift to her there—a stinky wet spot.

For two years after Kahlua died, Nikita was not himself. He too lost his sense of humor. He stopped taking a piece of turkey breast into the living room and growling at it as if it were a mouse, one of his favorite ways to get attention. In fact, this predatory instinct extended only as far as deli meats. Once, a real mouse ran across the kitchen floor, and Nikita merely turned his head to regard it nonchalantly. It scampered off, and Nikita made no move to chase it. Another time, a squirrel ran right across Nikita's tail. Then too he showed no interest.

Eventually, the passing of time healed Nikita's grief for his brother. Now, along with Lana, Nikita lives with Koshka, another longhaired Muppet look-alike. Both are Himalayans. Nikita is beige with brown ears and tail; Koshka is white with red ears and tail. Although they look alike, the two cats have never been close and have always just tolerated one another, both squished noses up in the air as they pass in the hallway. In terms of personality, Koshka is Nikita's opposite. Nikita prefers to pee on a rug; Koshka is meticulous about the box. Koshka loves to sit in the top level of his tall cat tree while Lana plays earthquake and rocks him to and fro; he likes to be jostled upside down and dropped onto the bed. He bats toys away in midair. During all these games, it's obvious that Nikita considers himself far too superior to play.

Lana missed Nikita's normal comical activities, which lightened her life so much. He was less likely to sleep in the crook of her elbow and knead her arm. When she took a bath, since Nikita had no fear of water, he would get into the bath too. Lana lifted him onto her chest, and he would stay curled up there for several minutes. Nikita liked big entrances and being the center of things. When he entered a room, he gave a chortle or funny meow to announce his presence and flicked the end of his uplifted tail. On floors, he would clomp, clomp, clomp his furry brown paws with the force of a tiny elephant. When Lana played the flute or sang, it always became a duet, because Nikita would yowl along with her, rubbing up against her leg. But now there were no games, no growling at deli turkey, no kneading, no bathtub invasions, and no smiles.

I had known Lana for over a year, because I had treated Nikita's back and hips using chiropractic and some acupuncture. Perhaps I should have known that his kidneys would be a problem because, according to the principles of Chinese medicine, the Kidney, hind leg mobility, and Bone are all intimately connected.

Lana's conventional vet and I worked well together, and via faxes, I found out that she had always been worried about his kidney function. After all, feline kidney failure is an epidemic in the United States! Holistic medicine places the blame on dry cat food, which is full of by-products and acts like a dry sponge that steals fluid from the body. We also blame overmedication, since the kidneys suffer the consequences of excreting potentially harmful drug metabolites from the body. Overvaccination can also harm the kidneys by plugging the nephrons with big antibody-vaccine complexes (see page 48).

Lana thought that Nikita's time was coming. One of the veterinarians at the emergency hospital had said that cats with kidney failure rarely gained weight again, and his words haunted her. "How did medicine become so negative?" I asked myself. She told me she was heartbroken to think she might lose her soft, longhaired friend. What would she do without his "Why bother taking things seriously?" smirk? Gathering all her remaining energy, Lana decided to file for an extension on the normal nine-life rule.

Lana brought Nikita in for me to begin aggressive treatment on his failing kidneys. While Lana recounted Nikita's story with the other veterinarian, the three of us hovered in a moment of despair. This was all such bad news. Nikita and I looked at each other. He had grown gaunt. But he still pawed at my arm as he always had, and in the blue of his eyes and the twitch of his pale whiskers, I still saw a hint of the unthinkable—a sense of humor.

For the first time in months, I heard my grandmother's voice loud and clear that day in the exam room with Lana and Nikita: "Focus on the positive. Look at everything that *is* working! Nikita's heart is good; his coat looks healthy; his liver is doing whatever livers are supposed to do." Grandma might have been sitting across from me during a family game of pinochle, secretly smiling, in her purple pantsuit and matching mauve sun visor. She never developed much of a poker face. It was as if, despite her crippling arthritis, she was beaming over a run and a hundred aces and was about to win the game for us. "And another thing"—Grandma was always one to speak her mind—"quit focusing on the poor fella's old kidneys!"

Grandma knew not a stitch of medicine, but she sure knew how to pick out the happiness amid the sorrow. She had a commonsense approach to life that I lost through years of studying medicine. Grandma would have agreed with the profound words of Gabriel García Márquez: "No medicine cures what happiness cannot."

It was almost as if Lana and Nikita felt my grandmother's ever-optimistic thoughts too, because at once there was a glimmer of hope on Lana's face. I thought of new treatment options and the three of us put our hearts into healing. I added vitamins to the fluids and instructed Lana on how to inject them under his skin, on his back, behind the shoulder blade. "He'll look like a hunchback for about twenty minutes," I told her, "and then he'll feel as good as new." Fluid therapy is good for flushing toxins out of the body and correcting dehydration. But it does nothing to strengthen the kidneys themselves—for that we needed acupuncture.

I started treating Nikita with Chinese needles into points known to strengthen kidney function. The tiny needles promote blood and nerve flow in the area of the kidneys. I also used moxibustion on certain acupuncture needles. Moxa would penetrate the body and strengthen it. Drawing upon the knowledge and treatments of many other holistic veterinarians, I prescribed Chinese herbs: two parts rehmannia 8 (Ba Wei Di Huang Wan) to ½ part Niu xu to strengthen the Kidney. These herbs have been used for thousands of years on people. For the past thirty years or so, holistic vets have been using the herbs for cats and dogs too.

During later treatments I added vitamin B_{12} injections in key "Back Shu" points that correspond to the Kidney and the Liver. I felt confident, because these injections, along with acupuncture, had helped many other cats deemed incurable by Western medicine, some of whom had creatinine at five to six times the normal level. Fluid therapy and other conventional medications alone had not helped these cats as much as when combined with holistic medicine.

Nikita's regular veterinarian had prescribed potassium pills and Lactulose for his constipation. A low potassium level in the blood renders cats' muscles weak and causes a reduced appetite, because it is a necessary chemical for muscle cells, even those of the intestines. Lana reported that indeed, Nikita seemed to perk up some, but he was still on a hunger strike. The fluids and potassium supplement helped Nikita come out from under the bed sometimes to take a little tuna water. I don't usually recommend tuna, but at this point, we were happy if Nikita ate anything.

He now stayed in the living room instead of hiding under the bed. His water consumption decreased a little, a good sign that he was better hydrated. But when Lana tried stirring the herbs into his food, boom! Nikita stopped eating again. She tried every trick in the book, and some new ones too, to get him to take the herbs: liver pellets, turkey jerky, Xodi's pet food garnishes, teriyaki turkey sprinkles, brewer's yeast. Her other vet suggested a local pharmacy that compounds any medication or herb into a number of different flavors. Fish oil, liver, and beef all resulted in different forms of feline rejection—foaming, gagging, or regurgitation—but tuna-flavored herbal medication led to just a little drool, qualifying it as a relatively successful endeavor. Lana had Nikita's sticky Lactulose and bitter potassium supplements compounded with tuna flavor too.

One month after we began treating Nikita, he was eating well and back to himself. He came in for acupuncture and fluid-therapy treatment once every two weeks. As with most cases, his holistic treatment was a group effort—everyone worked hard, even Nikita! According to Lana, he has always loved coming to my clinic, because I line my exam table with soft, fake-sheepskin covers and use aromatherapy, catnip, or whatever I need in order to relax the cats. I believe that cats have trouble recuperating in conventional practices partly because they're often stressed by cold steel tables, dogs barking, or the medicinal smell of anesthetic in the air.

One Saturday afternoon, in a deep gray Seattle winter, Lana brought Nikita in for his usual two-thirty appointment. She let him out of his carrier to explore my garden, behind the clinic. He came when she called him, to my surprise, turning down some fresh grass, and followed her into the clinic. His long white whiskers explored, his tail lifted; he had sticky patches of dried Lactulose on his otherwise well-groomed chest. He sat on my exam table as if he owned it, and I delicately placed the needles under his soft, long hair. The only movement he made was to place his front paw on top of Lana's hand, a ritual that has evolved over his thirty or so acupuncture appointments in the past year and a half. He did not cry or complain. In fact, he rested calmly for all but the fluid therapy, with a comical Wookie-like look that brought a smile to my face. It would be hard to take such a bulgy-eyed, furry face seriously, and he wouldn't wish it upon us to be so humorless. Like my grandmother, he had comedy in his blue eyes. He squinched his face tight and wiggled his ears at me. I could almost hear him laugh out loud. "Hey, he plays the water-bowl game again," Lana said happily.

Nikita's revival lifted my spirits. I keep a picture of him on my dashboard for emergency gridlock situations. I think my grandmother's sense of humor has become permanently part of who I am. I now practice seeing comedy in all things.

And there has been an unforeseen benefit to Lana's health as well. Nikita's improvement convinced Lana to go to an acupuncturist for her chronic fatigue syndrome. With diet changes, nasty-tasting herbs, and adrenal support through acupuncture, Lana feels much better. She found the strength to go to exercise classes and has much better endurance. Nikita is back to all his antics, eats well, and just had a birthday—he is seventeen years old and has gained two pounds.

⚘

Strategies for
Keeping Aging Pets Healthy

Many pet owners consider that ten to fifteen is old for a dog or a cat, but the world's record for the oldest cat is thirty-four years and for a dog, twenty-nine. Like people, as pets age they often develop more medical problems. The caseload for most holistic veterinarians consists of many geriatric animals. Acupuncture, gentle chiropractic, and many other holistic approaches will enable your pet to live out his golden years with fewer diseases and a lot less pain. The side effects from many medications, especially anti-inflammatory drugs, should be avoided, as those drugs are often harder on elderly pets.

I recommend that older pets eat homemade food (see diets, pages 28–30) with high-quality ingredients to preserve liver and kidney function. Because commercial pet foods tend to have by-products, rancid fats, and toxins from rendered animals, they do not necessarily promote longevity. Perhaps more important than cutting down on protein is to find more digestible protein sources, which many veterinarians are recommending. Homemade diets can do this beautifully, often giving the pet a new lease on life. People already feeding the BARF (bones and raw food) diet or other home-prepared foods to their pets will want to decrease the protein, as some diets call for up to 80 percent by volume of protein rations. My recommendation is that dogs should get at least one-third protein by volume throughout their life. Cats should get 50 percent protein by volume even as they age.

PREVENTION AND TREATMENT
OF COMMON AILMENTS

One of the most common complaints is that dogs, and to a lesser extent cats, develop cloudiness or a whitish haze in the pupils of their eyes. Your veterinarian may diagnose *lenticular sclerosis,* which does not cause the full opacity seen in cataracts. With this condition, pets still have vision, but their nighttime sight decreases. From a holistic standpoint, cloudiness is caused by excess liver toxins that accumulate over a lifetime. It can be treated with a homemade diet that includes freshly grated raw vegetables and the supplements mentioned earlier (see pages 28–30) and also a small amount of the liver-cleansing Chinese herb baical scullcap or huang qin (⅛ teaspoon a day for cats and ¾ teaspoon for a 50-pound dog). Some holistic vets prescribe bilberry (200 milligrams per 20 pounds of body weight) or grape seed extract (30 milligrams per 40 pounds) with the same goal in mind, that of aiding the body in toxin processing. It takes several months, and there is no guarantee, but I often do see an improvement.

Lipomas (fatty tumors), cysts, and warts are common in older dogs and should get checked at your veterinarian just to be sure they aren't some other tumor (malignant mast-cell tumors can mimic these benign growths). Lipomas indicate a stagnation of Qi and Phlegm in Chinese medicine terms. Usually they occur on the Gallbladder meridian, often on the same side as joint pathology, because it runs through the shoulders, hips, and knees. When there is stagnation in those joints, Phlegm coagulates elsewhere on the meridian. Blood and Qi moving herbs can help; acupuncture can also help. Most of the time, dogs develop these fatty tumors when fed commercial pet foods, which plug up the liver and gallbladder with toxins. Try a dairy-free, homemade diet and add turmeric powder (yes, the cooking herb, at 1 teaspoon per 20 pounds of body weight per day), which decreases inflammation in joints, supports the Liver, and moves Qi. Check with your veterinarian before using turmeric, especially if your pet is taking cardiac medication.

Stiffness, weak back legs, and arthritis are very common too as pets age. According to the principles of Chinese medicine, the Kidney controls the bone, opens into the ears, and gets damaged by fear. It is often the weakest meridian when the back legs get weak. Acupuncture or acupressure, massage, swim therapy, and a healthy diet are very important, as is regular exercise.

You can use glucosamine and chondroitin sulfate (250 milligrams daily for the average cat; 1,000 milligrams daily for a 50-pound dog), which, in a sense, replace the cartilage pets would get from eating bones. Glucosamine protects the cartilage within pets' joints and is very safe. I use a wonderful MSM/glucosamine supplement made by Frontier Herbs (see Resources, page 263) Some studies show that it helps prevent urinary tract infections too. Kidney support can be done with massage, herbs, acupuncture, and, in the winter, moxibustion.

Massage is a wonderful tool for helping all animals. *Four Paws, Five Directions* by Dr. Cheryl Schwartz has in-depth meridian diagrams and instructions, or consult with a T-touch practitioner in your area (see Resources, page 266). Basically, it can be done to relax muscles, stimulate acupuncture points, and help with circulation. Massage is crucial in pets with a deficient constitution, which often accompanies aging.

Massage Technique
Use the soft pads of your forefinger, middle finger, and ring finger and cup your fingers as if you are holding a steering wheel. Touch the animal with the opposite hand to "ground" him or her. Using the three-finger technique, in large, soft, slow circles work your way back toward the tail

from the head, along the pet's spine. You should not see that your nails get white from pressing too hard—the best technique is the softest.

The most important massage/acupressure techniques in aged dogs and cats are:

Stimulation of *Bladder 23*, "Kidney's Hollow," strengthens the Kidneys, especially Qi, Yang, and Essence. Use large clockwise circles, along the spine about one inch behind the last rib and about one inch on either side of the spine. This also benefits the ears (hearing is related to Kidney function), brightens the eyes, and strengthens the brain to aid in treating disorientation, lethargy, and a sensation of heaviness in the head.

Another important point to massage is *Stomach 36* ("Foot Three Miles"). The name describes its anatomical location in all species—three rib spaces below the knee, in the soft muscle belly. This point was commonly needled before a person embarked on a long journey because it is the master point for Qi and the Sea of Nourishment. It helps digestion, energy level, stiffness, and insomnia.

The final technique is a two-point hold on Kidney 3, the source point for the kidneys, and Bladder 60, the aspirin or alleviate-pain point. By some stroke of luck, these two points are located directly across from each other, so if you hold the web of skin just in front of the hock joint on each hind leg for thirty seconds or longer, you can stimulate both points.

Kidney 3, "Great Stream." The area between the medial malleolus and the heel tendon resembles a majestic stream; this point aids the Qi to flow through it. Tonifies the Kidney, source Qi, Blood, Essence, and warms Cold. By enriching the Yin, clearing deficiency Fire, and moistening Dryness, it helps constipation, red eyes, tooth pain, and lower-extremity numbness.

Bladder 60, "Kunlun Mountains." The name refers to the anatomy next to the lateral malleolus, which resembles a mountain. The Kunlun Mountains, in China, are considered the source of the Yellow River, where Chinese civilization began. Many philosophers, including the Taoists and Buddhists of ancient China, believed that mountains possess powerful energy and offer spiritual renewal. This point strengthens the back, relaxes the Sinews, facilitates Qi and blood flow, and helps ankle edema and pain.

THE MYSTERIOUS PAST LIFE
OF SHELDON T

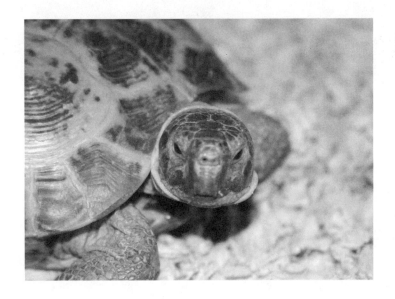

Craggled and wraggled and wrinkled. As round and grounded as our Mother Earth. My Russian tortoise is green and light brown, with beautiful, perfect rectangular patterns on his carapace—a wondrous, magnificent work of nature. He is simple, hardened, and tough but possesses the vulnerable and soulful wisdom of a hunched old man.

I watch Mr. Sheldon T's round shell meander across my lawn toward some scrumptious dandelions. He moves his head slowly from side to side, like a dinosaur, contemplating the terrain. All four of his sturdy scaled legs move beneath him. I wonder about his age—four or forty? Russian tortoises can live well over one hundred years. Who will I leave him to when I die? There's nothing like living with tortoises to make time seem infinite. Until recently, tortoises have been a successful species, spreading to every continent over the past five million years.

After I nursed my beloved Mr. Sheldon T back to health, after blood tests and radiographs and herbal teas, he disappeared one sunny day. He was in an enclosed pen outside; I turned my head for what seemed to be a minute, and that was when he vanished.

When tortoises really have a mission, they can scurry along fast. I combed the neighborhood, looking under bushes, in between plants and garbage cans, under rocks and grass clippings. After a few days, I decided at last to search underneath my neighbor's house.

My neighbor Lawrence is a loud-spoken, successful, and impeccably organized chiropractor who lives in a bright orange and green pumpkin house next to mine. He directed me to the small opening to the narrow crawl space under his house. "It's over there," he said, smirking playfully the way he did when I locked myself out. "If you crawl real close to the ground and slither along, eventually you'll get there." I knew that if Mr.

Sheldon T had reached the soft dirt, he would burrow underground the way he once did when he was wild, thousands of miles away.

I had second thoughts about exploring the dirty, dark space. But if Sheldon was under there, I couldn't just leave him. Besides, I needed to do penance for losing my beloved tortoise in the first place. So, wearing my dirtiest jeans, down I went, with a flashlight in one hand and a long stick in the other. Lawrence wished me luck and then drove off to work, leaving me alone to negotiate the dark.

I sank low, squeezing into the two-foot crawl space. As if I were moving clawed, stumplike appendages, I put one limb in front of the other. Arms and legs were buried in dirt, with only my eyes rising above the earth. I shone the light in search of the familiar round form, but I saw only rocks and pieces of insulation. It smelled like dirt, but with an odd hint of cleanliness and purity. "How could anyone have such clean-smelling dirt?" I wondered. My neighbor and I have always shared a lighthearted sense of competition, but in the category of tidiness, I am afraid I've lost. His house is planned via the laws of feng shui; mine, according to the laws of entropy.

Strangely, I felt safe there amid the sea of earth. Unaccustomed to the darkened underworld, I was surprised by how peaceful it was. There were no ringing phones or rumbling cars. The world was still. I could hear myself breathing. It seemed I had suddenly dipped deep into a meditative trance. Each of my limbs pushed dirt as I lumbered along. I felt as if I were part of the ground instead of towering above it, and I became aware of what life must be like tortoise style, closer to the pulse of our planet. How fitting that tortoises are the longest-lived vertebrates. It is as if they absorb and become part of ancient soils.

Millions of years ago, a protective armor offered great defense against the predators of that era. Tortoises and turtles were as successful as their dinosaur counterparts in a time when reptiles ran the planet. At New York's American Museum of Natural History, I remember staring in amazement at the two-million-year-old fossilized remains of an ancient tortoise, *Geochelone atlas,* found in India. He weighed over two thousand pounds and measured over seven feet in length. Long before the age of modern man, the giant tortoise ambled about seeking plants to eat. My much smaller six-inch Russian tortoises do the same.

Long after their fellow reptiles, the dinosaurs, became extinct, tortoises are still with us, but only barely. They have survived ice ages, but because of man, most of today's tortoises are endangered. They are still being taken from the wild, both illegally and legally, for the pet trade and for use in herbal medicine. Consumers should research tortoise ingredients in their Asian herbal medicine, like gui ban, or bie jia, or anything that says "shell" after it.

"It's no good," I said, wiping the soot from my mouth. I always talk to myself during stressful times. "I can't see him anywhere. I am the worst tortoise mom in the whole world." I felt sure I wouldn't find Sheldon. He had probably gone straight into hibernation, burrowing deep into the ground. I had let my little scaled friend down. I knew it was too damp for his frail shell outdoors in Seattle. Then there were raccoons and other potential predators. If only I lived my life more slowly, and did just one thing at a time, maybe I would not have lost him in the first place. Feeling a great sense of emptiness, I crept back up to the familiar world of light and noise.

Tortoises are much better adapted to the peaceful life of dirt dwelling than I am. Russian tortoises are outgoing, often stretching their heads and necks far out of their shells to say hello. When tortoises sleep at night, they let all four legs and head sprawl from their shells, eyes closed. Under wrinkly skin, the bones of their legs feel similar to ours—femur, kneecap, tibia, ankle joints, it's all there. They feel pain and I believe they also feel a whole range of emotions: stress, worry, jealousy, and affection. Russian tortoises blink just as we do, and when they open their relatively large mouths to eat vegetables, I see that their pink tongues look similar to mine. They are most at home living in their own burrows, but they are social too, often cohabitating. How different is my intermittent social life?

My first exposure to turtles was a brutal awakening. In college biology class, our teacher pithed (or killed by piercing the brain) a few in the name of proving some physiological law that to date I cannot remember. It was the only "fresh-kill" experiment I have ever experienced, having opted out of some in veterinary school. Since there were several students to each turtle, I did not participate. From the back, I could see the poor fellow getting dissected. It was awful, but I held it together for long enough to see his carapace split open, revealing a perfectly shaped Valentine's Day heart still beating faintly. With two atria on top and only one ventricle on the bottom, the reptilian heart is much more beautiful than the two-ventricle clump found within our own mammalian chests. I found it odd that the familiar

Valentine's heart shape so closely resembles the real heart of a reptile—an animal we have treated very poorly throughout history.

If I am honest with myself, I know that Sheldon always wanted to leave. Like the majority of Russian tortoises, he was captured from the wild to be sold in pet stores. In his case, I bought him at Petco. The day I picked him up, I felt bad for him. His shell was cracked, and a piece of it was missing. The salesman reassured me that he was domestically raised, but I researched and found out that, like other tortoises, Russians are very difficult to breed in captivity. Today there is little demand for domestic breeding, but there should be. In the year 2000, some 39,000 Russian tortoises were shipped out of Kazakhstan and approximately 35,000 each from neighboring countries, including Uzbekistan, Tajikistan, and Ukraine, to satisfy the pet trade. The United States imports more Russian tortoises than any other nation, closely followed by Japan. In fact, only 30 percent of the commercial demand in America for pet reptiles is met through domestic breeding.

These tortoises are listed as "vulnerable," which is the next category down from "endangered," and they're on the IUCN (International Union on Conservation of Nature) Red List 2000. This means that, due to this exploitation, a 20 to 50 percent reduction in the wild population is predicted over the next three tortoise generations. In contrast to the United States's open-commerce policy, Europe has voluntarily adopted legislation enforcing the recommendations of the Convention on International Trade in Endangered Species (CITES). Because of tortoises' poor survival rate during transport and in captivity, Europe has banned their importation altogether.

One conservation worker, who has since died in a land mine accident, witnessed the method by which Russian tortoises are "harvested" from Tajikistan. Paid the equivalent of only fifteen cents per tortoise, poor villagers collect them. The tortoises are then kept in large, overcrowded pens without food or water for up to seven weeks until the local "dealer" turns up in a truck. Then they are loaded into sacks, eighty to two hundred per sack, and shipped by road to the exporter, who is paid four dollars per tortoise. Not surprisingly, the U.S. importers and pet stores make the majority of the profit—up to one hundred dollars per tortoise.

Often, when we do buy a reptile, we do the poor creature an even further injustice by feeding it the wrong foods and ignoring the fact that it cannot maintain an adequate body temperature without external heat sources. The most common medical problem in reptiles is metabolic bone disease, in which their normally strong bones become as pliable as rubber. This is often caused by feeding meat to animals that are mostly, if not completely, vegetarian. The high level of phosphorus in meat, combined with the lack of calcium-rich leafy green vegetables, causes calcium to be leached from the bones. Sunlight is also required to activate vitamin D, another important building block for bones. Often, reptiles are deprived of sun, so special lamps are needed, especially during the winter. People often think of reptiles as "throwaway pets," and pet stores propagate ignorance by not educating people on how to feed and care for them.

When I found my tortoise at the pet store, he was knee deep in vegetable baby food; his shell was chipped and brittle. Because he was small and in less than perfect shape, I named him Mr. T, after the strong hero, to give him strength in the face of all his weaknesses. A friend thought the tortoise looked like a depressed poet, an existentialist author of sorts, so the first name Sheldon seemed appropriate. I fretted over the decision to buy him. I knew I would be part of the problem, buying him for half price, for only thirty dollars, with my Petco P.A.L.S. card, but I didn't realize how serious the tortoises' plight really was.

Everything seemed okay on the surface: Sheldon, me, a new leash for Sugar, all at the cash register at Petco. I didn't know that for every one tortoise that makes it alive to America, an estimated three more die along the way. They don't just softly expire either; instead, their brains, legs, and even perfectly shaped hearts get crushed in wood crates during transportation. They must struggle to survive, to breathe, and to avoid suffocation by another tortoise's blood. Many of them die slow, agonizing deaths.

All I could think of was the immediate gratification of seeing Sheldon heal, and I thought I could help him. Like many well-meaning pet lovers, I did not think of the big picture. Unlike my other tortoise, Igor, given to me years ago and generally relaxed in captivity, Mr. T was always looking over his shell to see if I noticed while he made attempts to hurriedly run away, to go home. I know that wild animals are best kept in their own natural setting; but now that he was loose, Sheldon risked acquiring shell rot from the damp climate here in Seattle. He was much better suited to the dry habitat of his homeland. But how safe was that homeland? Like much of the rest of the world, including America, the many nations around Russia see tortoises as expendable commodities. In his home country, if he dodged land mines and battlefields, he might be ground into fertilizer, a very common use for Russian tortoises.

After buying Mr. Sheldon T and monitoring him for illness, I noticed that his appetite dropped off and his stools became mucus coated. His shell was dull. I took him to Dr. Tracy Bennett, who took a small blood sample and radiographs, looking for infections or bladder stones. She also looked for parasites, which can be difficult to discover, in a stool sample. Many wild-caught tortoises have some parasites all their lives. According to Tracy, though, all the tests came back normal, so I decided to make Sheldon an herbal tea. I wished I could heal more than just Sheldon; I wished I could heal his whole threatened species, could provide a safe place for them to thrive, could end the pet trade that exploits them.

I wanted to use herbs indigenous to his Slavic home, but I didn't know of any. Instead, I collected devil's club, because of its deep spiritually and physically strengthening abilities; the Chinese herb isatis, cat's claw, pau d' arco, and other common immune-system tonic herbs. I sat on the couch with Mr. T in one hand and a small syringe of herbal tea in the other. After several minutes of failed attempts to pry his jaw open, I realized that he was more like an elderly man than I'd thought. Several years earlier, I had worked in a nursing home, and I remembered how difficult it was to convince old people to take their medicine. "Come on, Sheldon," I begged. "Please take a small bit." Nothing but a locked jaw and a stubborn wrinkled face stared back at me. Then I thought of a better way to get those herbs down him.

I took his favorite food, thawed frozen green beans, and wrung out the extra water. I sucked up some herbal tea with a needle and syringe and injected it into the shrunken green bean. I set it down in front of my stubborn tortoise patient. Suspicious, he turned to look at me, but I just pretended to fold some clothes behind him. It worked! Out of the corner of my eye, I saw him eat the fortified bean in two or three bites. The herbs worked their magic, and within just a day his stool was normal, resembling a Tootsie Roll. He became more active, following Igor in their large cage underneath the heat lamp.

Mr. T and Igor slept at night touching each other, their necks extended and heads resting on the floor. They were inseparable, often carefully and playfully nibbling on each other's noses, always touching or following each other. Baths were also a time of togetherness. Although they cannot swim, tortoises absorb enough water in shallow pools to hydrate themselves for several days. Igor happily gulped water with his mouth and low-

214

ered his nose beneath the surface while Mr. T lived up to his namesake, charging boldly toward the tumbling waterspout.

I couldn't expect Mr. Sheldon T to become very active. There is a slow steadiness in the tortoise world, a stable presence that exudes patience. In Chinese mythology, the tortoise symbolizes longevity, strength, and endurance. He is a messenger to the human race from the well-grounded Earth spirits. The *I Ching* describes a magic tortoise needing only sunlight and air to fulfill its needs. Native American folklore also recognizes the tortoise as Mother Earth herself, round and secure. Many tribes regard the tortoise as an island, with the ability to save drowning people and produce every living thing from its back. To the migratory Delaware Indians, the tortoise was important because they believed it preserved the land until they returned.

While Native cultures revered their indigenous tortoises, the European conquerors overharvested the giant tortoises as soon as it was discovered that these two- to six-hundred-pound giant creatures offered a fresh meat supply aboard ships. The ancient, giant tortoises were stacked alive on their backs and survived that way for months until they were eaten.

I will look for Mr. Sheldon T when the summer may awaken him from his months-long hibernation. My eyes will search constantly for movement in the grass amid the dandelions. I hope the herbal tea will fortify his hibernation, and I will not forget the lessons he taught me. We cannot speak of healing without considering the tortoise's life before the pet store. There are alternatives to propagating the wild-tortoise trade and there are a select few tortoise enthusiasts who have found the secrets to breeding them. We can make a collective decision not to buy wild-caught tortoises, and without demand, they will be left to their native lands. We can pressure the American pet industry to explore domestic rearing options. Perhaps we owe it to the tortoise to finally regard him with compassion and respect.

As we should safeguard each of our own individual histories by connecting with our ancestors, so too can we safeguard the planet by helping those ancient beings whose perfectly shaped hearts beat like Native drums. When we protect the wholeness of the tortoises' lives—caring for their physical bodies through proper husbandry and diet, treating their illnesses both holistically and conventionally, and ensuring their survival—only then can we pass on their long-revered, soulful lessons to our children:

Go slower.

Connect with Mother Earth.

Remember the past.

Caring for Your Reptile

Whatever you do, please find out about a pet instead of buying it on the spur of the moment. They are cute now, but they will grow! For example, a well-fed, healthy male iguana will grow to be up to six feet long including the tail.

It is obvious that reptiles are different on the outside from mammals, but they are even more different on the inside. Reptiles cannot control their own body temperature. Many of them are from warm places and need extra heat sources, especially in the winter. Be careful to find out what temperature is needed. Reptiles can burn themselves on hot rocks. Since they rely on sunlight to activate vitamin D, but are usually kept inside, a full-spectrum light is needed.

All reptiles have different heat and light requirements, so it is important to be educated about the particular reptile you are interested in. Also, each species may need special housing. For example, tree-dwelling lizards need branches and leaves to hide in. Diets are very specialized even between different tortoises; for example, some are desert adapted and eat dry, rough forage, while others are tropical and feed on lush leaves, fruits, and flowers. The horned lizard is insectivorous, primarily eating ants. Tortoises are mistaken for turtles all the time and kept in water, even though they don't know how to swim! You can buy a reptile from a breeder to make sure it is domestically bred. At this time, some snakes, certain lizards, and a few turtles and tortoises have been bred in captivity.

FOR WEBSITE INFORMATION ABOUT ALL SORTS OF REPTILES

www.kingsnake.com
    General information on reptiles and snakes.
www.anapsid.org
    This is Melissa Kaplan's care site. Her sections on diseases are
    extremely well researched and informative.
www.biology.Isa.umich.edu/research/labs/ktosney/file/BD.html
    This is Kathryn Tosney's site. She is a professor of biology at the
    University of Michigan. This site is great for information on
    bearded dragons.

CARE FOR RUSSIAN TORTOISES

Try to find a captive-bred or rescued tortoise by consulting the sources listed below. And don't do what I did and lose your tortoise! They are escape artists.

General information: Russian tortoises are six to eight inches long when fully grown and can live more than 150 years. The females are normally larger than the males. Carapace (top shell) coloration varies from light tan to yellow to olive, with brown markings. The distinguishing feature between males and females is the width and length of the tail—males have a bigger tail. Russian tortoises inhabit dry, barren localities. They normally hibernate most of the year by burrowing into mountain dwellings.

Diet: A high-fiber, low-protein diet is recommended. Eighty percent leafy greens: dark-leafed vegetation including nonsprayed grasses, clover, dandelion, mulberry, collard greens, and kale. Twenty percent other vegetables: lettuce (Romaine), peas, green beans, and tomatoes. They should eat at least every other day, but ideally daily owing to their herbivorous intestinal tract. There are mineral lotions that can be rubbed into their skin once a week.

Water: They don't need water in their habitat, as this can contribute to shell rot, and tortoises do not know how to swim! They absorb water through their skin, so mist them every other day in dry climates and soak them in a small amount of warm water (90 degrees Fahrenheit) for fifteen minutes at least twice a week. This will facilitate bowel and urate movements. They also get water from their food.

Temperature: The temperature gradient is important. One end of the habitat should be about seventy degrees and the other end about eighty-five degrees. Temperatures hotter than that may be dangerous. Remember that reptiles need you to regulate their temperature. Unlike mammals, they cannot do it themselves. Radiant heat sources are the best and safest. Ceramic heat emitters without a light can be left on all day. A low enough temperature slows the heart and may cause hibernation, but much research is needed to effectively hibernate a tortoise.

Lighting: They need a full-spectrum light or direct sunlight for about twelve hours a day. UVA/UVB light or, even better, sunlight is best. Turn it off at night. Tortoises perk up when they see light.

Bedding: I use Carefresh, a soft wood-pulp derivative. Alfalfa-pelleted bedding or "Bed a Beast" are okay too, but I am allergic to them. Tortoises love to burrow, and so some type of dirt substrate is okay. Bedding can be drying, so if you find your tortoise's skin peeling, be sure to soak or mist him more often.

Exercise: Allow tortoises to walk around very closely supervised. They love to walk. Don't leave them alone with your dogs!

WEBSITES REGARDING HUMANE TRANSPORT AND RESCUE INFORMATION ON TORTOISES

International Union on Conservation of Nature: www.iucn.org
Tortoise Trust Home Page: www.tortoisetrust.org
The New York Turtle and Tortoise Society: nytts.org
Hatchling Haven: home.earthlink.net/~rednine/
Turtle and Tortoise FAQ: www.tortoisetrust.org/care/faq.html
Chelonian-focused search engine:
    home.earthlink.net/~rednine/search.html
Graphic pictures illustrating immoral importation practices:
    home.earthlink.net/~rednine/cites.htm

WHITE POODLE BLUES

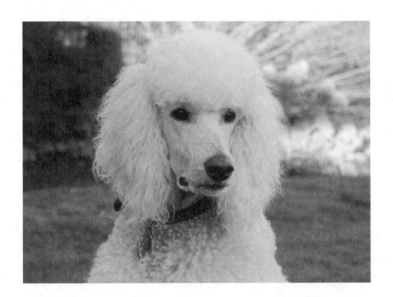

Despite his intelligence, charm, and intense good looks, Debby Dowd's white standard poodle, Jupiter, has always been a lemon. Almost from the moment she picked him up from the breeder, Debby noticed that young Jupiter didn't digest quite right. It was a fairly easy thing to overlook for a while, because Jupiter's thick white wool covered his thinning body and protruding ribs. Standard poodles are notorious for covering up illness, and Jupiter was no exception.

Chas and Debby are fifty-something intellectual types who research everything in life, including which breed of dog to choose. Chas's allergies led them down the hypoallergenic poodle road. In all honesty, Debby had wanted a mixed breed, but she reminded herself of what the books had said about standard poodles: smart, biddable, and calm indoors. Since then, she has become attached to both Jupiter, her white poodle, and Yankee, the black one.

Every time Jupiter received his recommended vaccinations, he vomited and had diarrhea all over their immaculate bamboo floors for several days. With each booster, his intestinal symptoms returned, intensifying, as if they were being driven deeper and deeper into his body. Of course, this association did not become clear to Debby until many months later. She was told that vomiting was normal for puppies, especially purebred, high-strung dogs, and since Jupiter was her first puppy, she had no idea what was normal. Over and over, she took his stool samples on the twenty-minute bus ride to the veterinary clinic for parasite analysis. She was sure that with enough testing, the vet would find a cause for his vomiting and diarrhea. With the determination that saw Debby through law school, she refused to give up on her pup.

Many dogs have transient problems after vaccination, but they are usually resolved after a period of time because the immune system is strong enough to correct itself. But for the weakest animals, this is not true. Jupiter's symptoms held on like ticks to rustling blades of grass. Not only that, they worsened with time, and soon Jupiter was vomiting for no apparent reason. Debby began to recognize the beginning of an onset of Jupiter's episodes; he would disappear from her side. When he was sick, she'd find him in a remote room of the house, standing in a corner with back arched, groaning, with an aching belly. He wouldn't eat for days and continued to have soft stools for months.

Debby was frustrated with the usual conventional treatments: Hill's bland intestinal diet (I/D), homemade chicken and rice, and holding Jupiter off food for twenty-four hours because nothing else helped. She was also tired of cleaning up after her poodle, and he, in turn, was embarrassed by his own mess. After all, he was a white standard poodle—a picture of perfection—and he *ought* to be clean and tidy. Debby switched vets and finally thought she had her answer. When the new vet, Dr. Donna Keirn, analyzed Jupiter's stool, she found two types of microscopic, one-celled parasites: cryptosporidium and giardia. But after several weeks on increasing medications, Debby reported that Jupiter's signs only worsened. Her hopes inflated and deflated like a balloon.

The outgoing Debby conferred with many folks about her dog, including a clerk at the local pet health food store who also happened to have a standard poodle, an epileptic who I was treating with acupuncture. The clerk suggested that Debby seek alternative medicine for Jupiter too. Acupuncture had treated Debby's tendon problems successfully, so why not Jupiter? she thought. She felt there were no other options left. Chas was upset too, and Jupiter's illness reminded him of why he hadn't really wanted pets in the first place. When Chas was small, his mother had found reasons to get rid of family dogs. Their disappearance had always been an emotional hardship, and now he worried about losing Jupiter.

Years later, Debby confessed to me that driving to her first acupuncture session, she questioned Jupiter in the backseat. "If you want to die, just tell me. I wouldn't keep you around just for me." She said he stared at her in the rearview mirror and made no overt answer. He just looked like his handsome self, peering back at her. With so many dreams for their dog-owner partnership, she was resolved to save him. There were tricks not yet learned, nursing homes gone unvisited, and obedience trials unattended. Debby dreamed as she worked away in her office/dog room that she would glance up and see Jupiter as he wanted to be—a normal, comfortable dog sleeping on his blue plaid pillow.

Before turning to acupuncture, Debby had tried many different diets and different veterinarians, and she was giving Jupiter twenty-four pills a day. Jupiter was taking several different antibiotics, antacids, steroids, and carafate. Cryptosporidium and giardia tests were still positive. He hadn't eaten for days, had daily uncomfortable episodes, and was thin. However, youth made up for his illness. Jupiter had not lost the spark in his dark eyes.

Dr. Donna Keirn is a very good doctor. We agreed that a simple case of parasitism should have cleared up right away. When intestinal problems worsen, more variables are involved. Normal or "healthy" bacteria help with digestion, and chronic antibiotic use kills them. The whole digestive tract suffers. The mucosal lining of Jupiter's stomach and intestines had been damaged over so many months of illness. Since vaccines may have triggered his intestinal woes to begin with, somehow his therapy needed to cleanse him of that damage. Little did I know that Jupiter would eventually help convince Dr. Keirn to take training in acupuncture and other holistic modalities. She was totally open to my intervention.

Debby brought Jupiter in, along with his long medical records from three different hospitals. He sat on the floor of my exam room, close to Debby. The poodle was meticulously cared for—his teeth were brushed daily and they were as white as his woolen coat. Looking back at that first appointment, I realize how sick Jupiter was.

At the time, I thought he should have looked worse, considering that he hadn't eaten for many days. If he avoided food altogether, he learned, he could avoid painful vomiting episodes. If Jupiter were a person, I could see him as a blond male model on the cover of GQ magazine. He was such a beautiful eye-catcher, and Debby groomed him in the newest poodle clips. And beneath his platinum ringlets, Jupiter was a standard poodle with emotional depth. He looked up at Debby, clearly worried about her.

Debby's features were sullen, her optimism tarnished by so many months of stress. Behind her eyeglasses, I could see dark circles, and I imagined that her gray hair was whitening even as we spoke. She reported everything to me, one symptom with each breath—the pain, the gas, the vomiting, the huge soft stools. "It's almost as if he can't digest anything anymore," she said. She was almost panting. Later she told me, "We are so much alike, Jupiter and I." She looked down at her beloved sick friend. "We both have intestinal problems and get anxious easily," she said, half smiling, self-consciously.

"The thing I can't understand," she said, releasing a long-standing worry, "is why we can't get rid of the giardia and the crypto. We don't go to any dog parks anymore." She sighed. "We can't even visit the nursing home because he might contaminate the residents."

"Well, maybe we need to focus less on the causative organism, or the bugs, and more on strengthening his digestive and immune systems. Parasites thrive in unhealthy bodies." I bent to look at Jupiter, who fluttered his lashes at me. I began my exam. Chinese exams are a little different from conventional ones. I looked at the dog's tongue to obtain information about its coating and color. It was pale and flabby and imprints of his teeth could be seen on the edges, where they pressed along its swollen border. The color of the tongue is important too—yellow indicates Heat, and white signifies Cold. Jupiter's tongue had a thin white coating. His ears and skin looked normal. But when I began to palpate under his stomach, he winced.

Pulse diagnosis is paramount in Chinese medicine, but I never feel I know enough about it no matter how much I study. It is a finely tuned skill that requires years to master. Still, I had to try. I placed my fingers softly on his femoral arteries, inside both back legs. "I'm learning pulse diagnosis, Debby, so have patience. This might take a while!"

"I have all the time in the world. I'm so worried about him," Debby said, stroking Jupiter's glamorous coat.

In Chinese medicine, there are many syndromes that can cause vomiting, weight loss, and diarrhea, and the pulses are the distinguishing factor. Blood swooshes through the arteries in different ways depending upon what is going on within the body. It can jump up to your finger with each beat of the heart, making it feel taut or wiry, indicating pain, or it can feel as if it's barely reaching your fingers; this is known as thready, and may show a body weakness. In Jupiter's case, the pulse was slippery—that is, it pushed against my finger with a quality that is said to feel like "pearls rolling around in a porcelain basin." Slippery pulses indicate an accumulation of Dampness within the body. The Dampness could be in the joints or other organs, but digestive symptoms usually indicate that this Dampness is coming from a weak Spleen. If there is one thing the Spleen doesn't want to be, it's Damp.

Each organ in Chinese medicine likes a certain climate. The Spleen likes hot and dry. In Seattle, we have too much dampness and cold, especially in the winter. I researched dietary causes for Dampness according to traditional Chinese medicine: fatty diets and alcohol. I pictured Jupiter out at bars while Debby and Chas slept, and somehow, I knew there must be another cause.

From the tongue and pulse, I knew there was Dampness accumulating in his system. Over time, this condition weakened the rest of the body, because the Spleen and Stomach are "the source of acquired constitution," or "Root of Postnatal Qi." Unless Jupiter lived in a plastic bubble, parasites would have set up shop. They prefer weakened bodies—and Dampness is like a nice petri dish for them. Maybe Jupiter was less of a lemon than we'd originally thought. His innate or congenital constitution might be weak, since he was a purebred, but the acquired portion, or what *we* did to him after birth, might be just as important. This includes over-vaccination and a diet of commercial pet foods. Besides, the acquired aspects of disease are the only things we can really control once the animal is already born.

The strategy would be to clear the Dampness and strengthen the Spleen. If my theory was right, the parasites would disappear along with the vomiting, diarrhea, and pain. Acupuncture could help right away, and I needled some points while we talked. Jupiter went right to sleep with the needles in place, which gave Debby and me time to discuss possible causes of his condition from a holistic point of view.

There are many factors important for good digestion, and all of them have to work together like a huge digestive orchestra. The vagus nerve and other parasympathetic nerve impulses control peristalsis, or gut motility, and secretions must be functional. Stress interferes with vagal impulses and this explains why stress affects digestion.

Correct nutrition is vital too, although there is much discussion as to what exactly "correct" is. Beyond protein, carbohydrate, fats, and vitamins, there are several other often-forgotten factors. A balance of good intestinal bacterial flora is necessary to break down food. Adequate pancreatic enzymes and bile are needed to aid in the absorption of fine food particles. The acid/base balance must be maintained. The stomach is very acidic, but within the intestinal lumen there is less acidity as the food moves farther down the intestinal tract. Toxins from other organ systems, such as the Liver or Kidney, may cause digestive problems if those systems are failing. Even in conventional medical terms, the number of variables that affect digestion is mind-boggling.

Chinese medicine considers all these variables, with the addition of patterns such as a deficiency or stagnation of Qi, Phlegm, Blood, and an accumulation of Dampness and Phlegm. All can affect digestion. In Chinese and Ayurvedic medicine, temperature differences are a big factor in digestion. Fatty diets cause a buildup of "ama," to use an Ayurvedic term, causing toxic reactions in many body systems. It's so complicated that it's amazing more pets don't have digestive problems.

How do vaccines relate to all of this? Well, in homeopathy there is the principle of miasms, which contends that the body holds on to certain events and substances in specific weakened organs. Later in life, disease may result in the same body systems that were originally affected. Many of the viral pieces contained in the routine five-way vaccine for dogs are intestinal in origin. I believe that the local intestinal antibodies and other inflammatory cells create weakness in the gastrointestinal tracts of some dogs after they are vaccinated.

The energetic propensity to hang on to that vaccine-induced intestinal stagnation causes Dampness, especially in dogs with a constitutional propensity toward it and the genetic inability to compensate for it. This includes purebred dogs and cats but can occur in any animal. These weakened animals would be more inclined to develop food allergies later in life, because even for many years following vaccination, inflammatory cells and local antibodies are easily triggered, like soldiers guarding the intestinal wall from foreign invasion. The confused immune system believes food to be the archenemy—setting up chronic intestinal inflammation. With all the immune system's attention on the gastrointestinal tract, other bodily organ systems may be more prone to infection.

The other danger of chronic Dampness or intestinal inflammation is the possibility of later developing intestinal cancer. Generally, vaccines do their job—they prevent certain viral infections—but for Jupiter, especially in their repetition, they also caused unwanted side effects. By now Debby and Jupiter were just about sleeping in the corner of my exam room. I had thought about the poodle's intestines enough, and now we needed a game plan. "Let's take him off the antacids and antibiotics and just keep him on carafate, because it is like an intestinal Band-Aid," I said. I like to use herbs with soothing effects similar to those of carafate, but that provide even better mucosal healing and nutritional properties. We could start Jupiter on slippery elm and marshmallow root when his carafate ran out.

Jupiter took well to acupuncture. I needled points such as Stomach 40 ("Abundant Flowering"), a phlegm-clearing point just below each stifle, and Spleen 9, on the insides of both hind legs. I used Bladder 20 ("Spleen's Hollow"), which is located on either side of the spine in front of the eleventh rib in dogs and cats. It is the Spleen association point, and controls the spinal nerves flowing to the pancreas. Conception Vessel 12 ("Middle Stomach Cavity") is a point on the belly some dogs don't like, but Jupiter didn't mind. He slept while Debby and I talked.

"Whether Jupiter heals himself or not depends almost as much on what you do at home as what we are doing here," I said. "A home-prepared diet is really important." Debby nodded.

In general, commercial pet food is not good for dogs with intestinal sensitivities, for several reasons. The texture of kibble is dry and irritating to mucosal surfaces, and both dry and canned food often contains unhealthy ingredients. The most damaging of them may be rendered animal meal. Because the preparation of commercial pet food is largely a self-regulated industry, many unsavory and even deadly ingredients may be included. According to the FDA, this food can contain pentobarbital, a deadly chemical we use to euthanize animals. In 2001, the FDA admitted that traces of it survive the rendering process and enter pet food. Says the FDA's Don Aird, "We had reports from vets that dogs had died after eating foods that contain pentobarbital." Even though the Pet Food Institute denied using rendered dogs and cats, it is being done on a regular basis. Aird said that if pet food were eaten by people, there would be an immediate recall. Some "natural" brands of dog food probably do not contain rendered products. It is not yet public which brands contain pentobarbital and which do not.

I know Debby didn't want to hear about the commercial pet food controversy, and I didn't want to talk about it. But of course, I had to, for Jupiter's sake. I wrote down a diet for Debby to make at home. Whereas conventional vets like to limit the number of foods, holistic vets often wish to increase the variety. If food allergies are part of the picture, shifting foods can alleviate them. I knew the poodle was too weak to handle raw diets, so I prescribed a cooked diet of organic turkey, yams, a few sardines, oats, and spinach, plus vitamins and enzymes. Jupiter soon became known as "yam man" at Dr. Keirn's office.

"If Jupiter's belly ever gets big and tight, it's a condition called bloat, and it's an emergency," I said. "It is common in large, deep-chested breeds, especially Great Danes, but I have seen it in standards, so I just want you to be aware of it."

"What causes bloat?" she asked. "How can we prevent it?"

"Well, in Western medicine, no one can say for sure. It is sometimes brought on by changes in food or some other underlying disease like cancer. There could be an unknown nutritional cause. A recent study from Purdue University showed a possible association between feeding foods containing citric acid and the incidence of bloat. Many times it is very difficult to be certain of the precise cause. The stomach twists and flips over, making it impossible for the dog to vomit. Depending upon the severity of the torsion, veterinarians may be able to pass a stomach tube down the esophagus and pump the stomach. If the tube fails, emergency surgery is needed to suture the stomach in place," I said, stopping to check on Jupiter's needles. "I think natural diets and acupuncture can really help prevent it, but I just want to make you aware of it."

Jupiter improved somewhat after our first treatment. As I suggested, he was eating very small amounts several times a day. I also suggested that Debby replace the carafate with a gruel of slippery elm, marshmallow root, and fennel, which she had to syringe into Jupiter's mouth between meals. Later, she confided that this was no easy task, owing to her poodle's lack of cooperation. Both she and Jupiter became soaked with herb-tainted liquid until she learned the cardinal rule of giving obstinate pets medication—don't stand in front of them. Once Debby learned to straddle the dog and squirt the gruel in from the side, things went better.

The most amazing achievement was that not only did he begin to eat again, but generally, he kept most meals down. Over the next several months, Jupiter continued to improve, but he still had episodes of pain—standing in the corner cramping and vomiting. I prescribed at least ten different herbs to help digestion and gave him several dozen acupuncture treatments and occasional chiropractic. Jupiter was still eating the homemade food and keeping it down between episodes. He was off all conventional medication, and fecal tests showed that he was finally clear of both crypto and giardia infections.

Jupiter was better, but not cured. If we did acupuncture every week or two, he was symptom-free, but the minute we tried to decrease the treatments, some of his original symptoms returned. He was still thin. Then I took the NAET course in California and decided to try it on Jupiter.

NAET, Nambudripad's Allergy Elimination System, was developed by Dr. Devi Nambudripad, who uses a combination of chiropractic and acupuncture to treat allergies. The technique helped my own allergy-based asthma, which I have always struggled with. Unfortunately, I am allergic to dust, cats, and horses—it's surprising how many veterinarians develop allergies to animals. Mine have been bad my entire life, because the lung is my weakest organ. Jupiter's weakest system is his gastrointestinal tract. Allergies cause Dampness, which often collects in our weakest organs. For me, the allergen might be cat fur, and for Jupiter, it might be foods. In either case, the immune system's recognition process is not normal. Instead of attacking only viruses and bacteria, it attacks the wrong things.

Debby met the whole notion of NAET with resistance at first. "I know Jupiter was improving with just the acupuncture and diet, and now I know he has stagnated. But this whole NAET thing is just crazy," she said. I didn't blame her, because I had felt the same way until I saw it clear allergies firsthand. I had to resort to begging Debby to try the new-fangled technique. Perhaps because it was pathetic to see a grown veterinarian groveling, she consented. "But we can't tell Chas, not unless it works," she whispered.

"Mum's the word," I promised, thrilled because I knew that, like acupuncture, NAET was extremely safe. While NAET doesn't work with every allergic animal, I knew it could bring patients through a therapeutic plateau—when they have improved as much as they can with acupuncture and herbs. Many times clients won't take chances without a guarantee, but Debby and Jupiter hung in there with me.

The idea with NAET is to individually test foods, vitamins, and environmental allergens using a special kit. This kit looks similar to the one an allergist might use to inject small amounts of an antigen to look for a reaction on the skin. The difference is that with NAET, rather than injecting potential allergens into the body, the patient touches the vial with one hand while the practitioner tests muscle resistance on the other—this is called contact reflect analysis, or muscle testing. When a particular vial causes a problem, the patient's muscles grow weak, so the practitioner can more easily push his arm down. Many common foods are tested, such as eggs, vitamins C, A, and B, sugar, and grains.

With regard to animal patients, NAET muscle testing must go through a surrogate, or the owner of the animal, since obviously we can't directly muscle-test animals. This is perhaps the hardest part about the treatment to accept. The person holds a vial, say of vitamin C, on the dog's skin and the practitioner tries to push her other hand down. If her hand is weak and she is unable to hold it up, her dog is allergic or does not process the vitamin C properly. Essentially, there is an electrical circuit between the practitioner, person, and pet.

As you may have guessed, Jupiter was allergic to almost every basic food. One by one we cleared them, using NAET. "Clearing" is the therapeutic part of treatment, in which the allergenic vial is held on the animal for twenty minutes while the doctor uses a specific combination of chiropractic and acupuncture or acupressure. This treatment energetically tells the body not to react to the allergen but to incorporate it into the "normal" energetic sphere. After a treatment, the patient should avoid the substance for a full day to give the immune system time to shift.

Every week, Jupiter plopped down in the middle of my clinic carpet while Debby touched him with one hand and held her other hand out to the side. We held different foods, treats, and supplements up to his skin, and I would try to push Debby's arm down. The cool thing about muscle testing is the mutual understanding between the animal's owner and the practitioner. In other words, Debby could tell which vials and foods were a problem for Jupiter simply because they would weaken her arm. This form of treatment empowers clients and deepens the connection with their pets, because the human clients are such an important part of the process.

It took about eight clearing appointments to see that his vomiting sessions were diminished. The thin, narrow-chested dog we once knew as Jupiter was transformed over a few months. Instead of a gaunt male model, Jupiter became as robust and muscular as Brad Pitt. Although Debby and I are not sure the white poodle will ever have a completely normal digestive system, we continue to marvel at his progress. It's been six months since he vomited, and he even raided the garbage recently. Debby and Chas rejoiced because it did not make him sick. Jupiter goes places now. In fact, he just received his AKC champion dog title in obedience!

What to Do for Digestive Trouble

Dogs with indiscriminate appetites who get into garbage may develop vomiting and diarrhea. Cats vomit very easily, so occasional vomiting and diarrhea, say once a month or so, is normal, especially for an impeccably self-groomed, long-haired cat who develops hairballs.

HOW DO I KNOW WHEN MY PET NEEDS CONVENTIONAL CARE?

- Any young puppy or kitten with vomiting, diarrhea, or loss of appetite may have an infectious disease or a vaccination reaction.
- Vomiting often, especially if the animal can't keep food or especially water down, or continuous diarrhea.
- Vomit is pink tinged or diarrhea contains large amounts of blood or mucus. If the stool is black and tarry, this may be digested blood.
- Animal acts depressed or lethargic.
- Pet tries but cannot vomit or defecate, or the abdomen appears swollen; this may be GDV or bloat. Go to vet at once! Emergency!

There are many intestinal diseases that need conventional care, including acute pancreatitis, foreign body obstruction, and poisonings.

USEFUL CONVENTIONAL TESTS AND TREATMENTS

Perhaps the most important question when deciding whether or not to do diagnostic tests is: Will the test have an impact on the treatment? Sometimes vets do tests because we are good at tests, but do not spend all your money on tests and have none left for treatment.

- Fecal analysis to check for parasites and deworming, especially in young animals.

231

- Blood work to check conventional liver, kidney, and other vital parameters. Remember that there often needs to be a 70-percent reduction in organ function for the blood to show problems.
- Abdominal radiograph or ultrasound to see foreign objects blocking intestines, congenital malformations, or tumors.
- Antibiotics are often beneficial when intestinal villi have been damaged.
- My least favorite drug is the overprescribed metoclopramide (Reglan), because it suppresses vomiting and can often cover up severe disease. Used discriminatorily, it can be very effective for certain diagnosed pathologies.
- My favorite conventional intestinal soother is carafate or Sucralfate, because it is safe and effective, but see herbal options below.

Hooray for Conventional Fluid Therapy!

Fluids are by far the best thing Western medicine has given to dehydrated animals who suffer from ongoing vomiting or diarrhea. Fluids correct water and electrolyte losses.

HOW DO I KNOW WHEN MY PET COULD BENEFIT BY HOLISTIC CARE?

- When all other tests do not explain digestive symptoms.
- Pet feels sick for a few days after vaccines.
- All conventional treatments have not helped or the pet cannot tolerate the side effects of medication.

NATURAL GUIDE FOR VOMITING/DIARRHEA

- Hold off food for twelve hours. Give one of the homeopathic remedies listed below or *Nux vomica* 30C just once during this tummy-resting period, but give plenty of water or broth.
- After twelve hours, give him a digestion-soothing, bland diet, a small amount with frequent feedings. Small dogs: ½ cup cooked brown rice, ¼ cup cottage cheese, homemade or low-sodium chicken broth. Large dogs: 2 cups cooked brown rice, ½ cup cottage cheese, homemade or low-sodium chicken broth. Cats: ⅛ cup cooked brown rice, ¼ cup cooked white-meat chicken or fish.

- If successful, continue diet for two to three days before introducing pet to any commercial pet food. If symptoms return when commercial food is added, this is a sign that your pet's diet may be a potential cause of irritation.
- If animal's symptoms return, try the herbal tea below, which can heal intestinal mucosa. This tea could also help after intestinal surgery, when the animal is eating again.
- I do not recommend herbal parasite treatments without professional care, because herbs powerful enough to kill parasites can be toxic to pets.

Colic Remedy

Combine 1 tablespoon of fresh dill with 1 teaspoon of gingerroot and 1 cup of hot water. Allow it to cool to body temperature before dosing. Many European veterinarians use it for horses with gas colic. For dogs and cats, use the same dose as Intestinal Healing Gruel, below.

Intestinal Healing Gruel

1 cup low-sodium chicken broth or water
3 tablespoons dried cut marshmallow root (or 2 tablespoons powder)
3 tablespoons slippery elm bark (or 2 tablespoons powder)
1 tablespoon dried meadowsweet leaves (or ½ tablespoon powder)

Combine all of the ingredients in a stainless steel or ceramic saucepan, cover, and simmer over low heat for 20 minutes, taking care to replace the broth or water to the original level if there is evaporation. Remove from the heat, uncover, and let cool and sit for about 6 hours. The tea should be slimy because its mucilaginous consistency acts like an intestinal Band-Aid. Give 1 teaspoon to cats twice a day with a turkey baster or syringe. Give 1 tablespoon per 25 pounds body weight for dogs. It is safe at almost any dose, even with other medications and over prolonged periods of time.

Keeping: The tea will last for just 1 week in the refrigerator.

None of the herbs is antimicrobial. Unlike other herbal teas, it shouldn't be frozen, because some of its slimy active ingredients may get destroyed. Bring to room temperature before using.

TRY HOMEOPATHY

If symptoms are ongoing and herbs do not help, homeopathic remedies are available at health food stores, natural pharmacies, or homeopathic distributors (see page 263). Homeopathic remedies are safe to give along with conventional medications but please go to your veterinarian whenever there is repeated vomiting or diarrhea.

Nux vomica 30C, a.k.a. colubrina, will help indigestion when it has been caused by eating rich food (sweets, cakes, chocolate bars). It will be more effective when there is frequent vomiting and listlessness.

Bryonia 30C may also be helpful for indigestion when the pet does not want to eat, seems to have a bellyache, and stays for a long time in the same spot.

Pulsatilla 30C should be the choice when the indigestion was caused by fatty/greasy food and the pet follows you around and whines or pants.

RIO'S RIVER OF QI

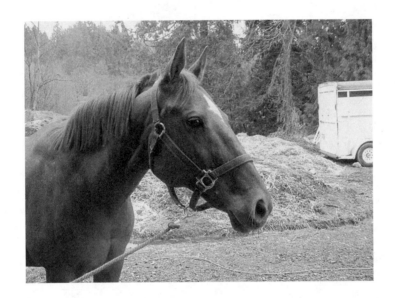

Two Tuesdays a month, at about twelve noon, I have a date with a chestnut mare named Rio. She is lucky enough to live at one of the last remaining stables with acres of rolling green pastures in the growing Seattle suburb of Redmond.

On the way to her stall, I pass all her stable mates. At horse stables, when you have an appointment with one horse, you come to know the other horses too, as if by osmosis. There is the darling, ever-assertive Oreo, a black-and-white-splotched pony who, like most ponies, is used to getting whatever he wants. And the sensitive, easily offended big gray mare named Sasha, who kicks her stall violently when you don't greet her properly. As soon as you regard her politely, from the front of her stall, she nuzzles your palm sweetly. And Snoopy, a pretty bay hypochondriac who is sure that not only will he die within the next few minutes, but it'll hurt too. Without the confident and dependable Rio, Snoopy would shudder with panic attacks even more than he does now.

There's no doubt that Rio is the levelheaded one of the bunch. I wouldn't consider Rio to be an especially fancy horse; she is certainly no imported Hanoverian or Arabian. Susan Cole, the barn manager, found her in the *Little Nickel* classifieds. She had no papers and Susan knew nothing about her history. But Rio won Susan over, because the horse is as pretty as she is even tempered. One notices the wide diamond-shaped star on Rio's forehead, and her bright orange sleek coat, not her portly barrel.

Munching on hay, she calmly comes over to say hi. She pricks her ears and opens her large dark eyes wider to greet me. I place my hand on her forehead. With their complex social skills, horses need touch, and they learn from it. Without knowing it, humans convey all sorts of information about themselves to the horse just through simple contact. Perhaps it's the pressure of my hand or some psychic force in the patient, but I know that Rio picks up on my intent, my level of ability, and my kindness.

Rio and I have come to know each other well over the course of a year of visits. You might say we have an ever-evolving, deepening respect for each other. We probably wouldn't have chosen each other's friendship under other circumstances. I'm usually partial to horses who, like myself, are spontaneous and fiery. Likewise, Rio might have chosen a human friend more like herself—surefooted and more considerate.

Rio's relationship with her pasture mates, especially Snoopy, has always been curious to me. I've always wondered what sends Snoopy into such fits of panic and what it is about Rio that calms him. Being an ex-racehorse, Snoopy may be neurotic due to the track experience or just because he's a thoroughbred. To Snoopy, every windblown leaf or innocent barn swallow is a potential suspect, along with everything else that twitters or moves suddenly. For him, bush monsters lurk at every edge of his pasture, falling tree branches are just camouflaged nuclear warheads, and the evil, two-toed, red-eyed green dragon is just waiting behind the next corner to devour him.

When Snoopy's panic attacks hit, his nostrils flare, his head goes up, his eyes open wide, and his big dark bay body seems to swell to twice its normal size. He shakes all over and explodes like a bomb, trying to gallop away even if he's tied up. Rumor has it that these episodes were an almost daily event before Rio arrived. Now, Snoopy stays nuzzled up to her like a baby: She is his security blanket. Rio seems to know her newfound importance in the world. She wiggles her muzzle on Snoopy's back, and the two horse friends can often be seen scratching each other's withers with their teeth.

When Susan Cole first called me, Rio had developed a sarcoid on the corner of her right eye. The most common skin tumor in horses, sarcoids are not metastatic—that is, they don't spread—but they are locally invasive and can grow to be big and deep. Among horse people, sarcoids are well known and frustrating. Frequently, they return, after conventional intervention, and return with a vengeance, often growing faster and bigger than before.

Rio's regular veterinarian had told Susan that there were essentially two options: surgery or injection. Surgery would leave a nasty gaping wound, and injection would likely cause tissue death around the tumor, otherwise known as "sloughing." We all worried about the sensitive location of the tumor. With conventional medicine, damage to the tear ducts was to be expected. Eventually, Rio's eye might have to be removed.

The specific cause of sarcoids is unknown, but the list of potential culprits includes genetic predisposition, viruses, and previous trauma to the tumor site. Many therapies have been attempted, yet none is routinely successful. With each therapy, about 50 percent of the tumors recur.

Susan was also told that occasionally sarcoids do regress on their own. But seemingly with each passing day, Rio's sarcoid doubled, then tripled in size. In just a few weeks, it grew to occupy the entire inside of the eyelid. "Such a shame to lose a perfectly good eye," Susan said, obviously worried, when we first met.

From the start, I did not think holistic medicine would shrink the sarcoid, but Susan never lost faith. Susan has been around horses all her life. She assumed that if we could clear Rio's body of toxins and do acupuncture to allow the energy to flow smoothly, the sarcoid would vanish into thin air! I thought this was wishful thinking, but I agreed to try. Although I always try to remain positive, I couldn't help thinking we would be lucky to stabilize the mass. I found Susan's power of positive thought, her overriding belief that we would win, a little hard to believe.

It is said that the body's life energy force, its Qi, flows like water. The acupuncture points on the ends of fingers and toes are called "Jing well" points, because the energy bubbles up from them as water might from a small but powerful underground spring. Each point along any meridian opens into wider and wider channels, like a river courses to the ocean. This is why many of the more powerful Qi directing points are located toward the extremities of the body. How appropriate that *rio* means "river" in Spanish. Every time I saw the chestnut mare, I imagined Qi flowing through her body, overcoming barriers the way a flooded river bypasses a dam.

Rio's river had so many dammed up, blocked areas. The first thing I noticed was that her sarcoid had formed at the acupuncture point Stomach 1. This meridian ends at the front of the back hoof, and curiously enough, Rio had a large scar directly on Stomach 45, the last point on that meridian. Perhaps her sarcoid was a simple blockage of energy. Wounds and scars can act like a cage and trap the Qi within a channel. In addition, all Rio's extra weight was going to her belly—the first time I saw her, I thought she was pregnant—whereas her topline was thin. This can be another symptom of Qi Stagnation. It can also mean only that horses are out of shape, just like people.

Growing up with horses, I learned about strange diseases particular to the equine, such as sweeney (a shoulder disorder caused by nerve damage and muscle atrophy), stringhalt (a neurological condition in which the horse involuntarily lifts a hind leg), and strangles (a strep infection that causes yellow nasal discharge). I had always heard the traditional horse-related old wives' tales, some true and others more far-fetched. For example: "Don't tie a horse you don't know." (Horses can injure themselves trying to get free.) "Never let a sweaty horse drink before cooling him off." (Horses can colic from drinking too much or from "tying up," a condition in which the muscles become rigid and painful.) "Chestnut horses are the most sensitive." I hadn't given this one too much thought, but as I came to know Rio, it seemed to ring true.

At first I used Dr. Are Thorensen's famous "Control, or Ko Cycle." This approach to treating tumors strengthens one acupuncture point with the purpose of supporting the Gallbladder, which controls the stomach. Initially, I used Gallbladder 44 ("Foot Yin's Aperture"), a point just above the hoof on each hind leg, as well as Stomach 2, a point just below each eye. (The latter's Chinese name, "Four Brightness," refers to the point's function of enabling one to see in all four directions with renewed clarity.)

Owing to Rio's trust in people, she let me needle almost any point easily. It was remarkable. Qi flowed so easily that within minutes after each treatment, Rio's large brown eyes glassed over. She chewed without food in her mouth, another sign of relaxation in horses. Why was Rio so relaxed about life when her horse buddies panicked at invisible monsters? Susan always says that Rio is savvy, that she's one of the few horses that would survive in the wild. "She's just confident about where she fits in the world," Susan said one day as we watched the chestnut mare rest in the aisleway with her needles.

Susan and I noticed that the growth of the sarcoid, which had been fast, was now slow. I prescribed blood-moving Chinese herbs, but I worried that it would cost too much to get enough herbs into Rio's food. We tried using many topical treatments on the tumor. It was difficult, because we had to be careful not to hurt the eye. We used comfrey on the ulcerated, bleeding areas, and thuja oil, which is usually used for warts. Busy barn manager that she is, Susan found shortcuts for these treatments.

"Why does Rio have duct tape on her face?" I asked one Tuesday. Rio seemed a little embarrassed about the tape, but it didn't hurt her; it barely stuck to her hair.

"That's how I do the comfrey poultices," Susan giggled. She always had such a good sense of humor.

Months passed with little change in the sarcoid size. We were happy that it hadn't grown but still disappointed that there had been no improvement. Rio was happy, though, and lived her normal pasture-roaming life, keeping Snoopy sane just by staying close to him. She was a horse burdened with many responsibilities.

One day, by chance, her regular veterinarian and I were at the stables at the same time. That day, we all stood around Rio's eye, trying to judge the size of her sarcoid. "It looks bigger," I said. The more I stared at the ugly, ulcerated mass, the larger it seemed.

"I think so too. You know, the longer we wait on injecting it, the harder it might be to finally shrink it," Dr. Brookfield said. I knew she was right, though it was hard to admit defeat.

"No," Susan said, "I'll try another herbal salve. It still isn't bothering her. Let's wait." I wondered how long it would be before Rio would have trouble producing tears, or even seeing past the lump. For now, it was true, rather than rubbing her eye on the wall, Rio didn't seem the least bit concerned about her sarcoid. The conventional vet and I agreed to wait.

Animals can tell when we are worried about them—when we fundamentally believe that they will not be okay—and it causes them stress. Instead of turning their healing abilities inward, they expend vital energy in worrying that we are worrying. Often the best thing we can do is tell them that it is not so bad. I overheard Susan speaking to the chestnut mare: "Rio, I know you have an ugly tumor, but you know we all have some problem or another, and besides, it's going to get better." The horse pricked her ears forward to listen intently.

After her vet left on another call, Susan and I sat side by side on a hay bale, trying to decide what to do. We looked at the ingredients in her tumor-eating salve: bloodroot and zinc chloride. "This stuff is going to slough that tumor off," I told her. "It might really hurt the eye too if it oozes accidentally beneath the lid," I said. We pondered this dilemma for many minutes.

I couldn't help remembering years earlier when I worked as a riding instructor. One of our old school horses developed a sarcoid on the right side of his face—a common location—and also on the Stomach meridian. The veterinarian did surgery after surgery, leaving a larger and larger wound. It was really disgusting looking, and I felt so bad for the horse. He grew wary of people and seemed to be in so much pain.

I decided to move into sarcoid-fighting overdrive. If Susan wouldn't give up, then neither would I. "Let's try changing the acupuncture points and do some NAET," I suggested. (See page 229.) I added many more points, realizing that Rio's tumor was also on the upper lid, close to Bladder 1. I used Dr. Thorensen's approach (Large Intestine 1 above the inside front hooves), as well as points Stomach 40 and Bladder 40—Baiwai that move Phlegm and stagnant Qi—according to Chinese medical principles. For an hour, Rio stood patiently while the needles worked.

The next week, I brought my NAET vials and discovered that Rio was allergic to minerals and grains. Could these allergies be causing stagnation along the Stomach meridian too? We cleared her for these allergies. At about the same time, Susan began massaging Dynamite Wound Balm into a huge knotted scar on Stomach 45.

Within a few weeks, Rio's sarcoid had shrunk visibly, although Susan and I wondered if we were imagining it. Poor Rio peered at us as we stared at her eye—how strange we must have looked to her, with Susan lifting her eyeglasses and me squinting, both within inches of her face. If we did upset her, she never let on. Indeed, Rio seemed happy to chew on her hay while we performed our regular inspections.

I am not sure if it was shrinking Rio's scar at Stomach 45, using NAET to help with food allergies, treating her with acupuncture, adding antioxidants to her diet, or a combination of all these things, but today, one and a half years after I began treating Rio's sarcoid, she is much better. The tumor is gone. (To see Rio's tumor shrink, go to www. wholepetvet.com.)

We don't know what the future will bring; the tumor could come back. Skeptics would probably say what they usually say in these situations: "Well, that tumor would have gone away by itself." I don't know about you, but I rather doubt it. For me, Susan's power of positive intent rang true. And now she's on emergency tumor alert—if the sarcoid grows even a tiny bit, she'll call me right away. If not, then Rio can carry on, calming Snoopy down and watching out for all the other horses—watching with both eyes.

Holistic Care for Horses

Horses are such amazing creatures, but, as we breed for speed or personality, we are forgetting a very old English proverb, "No foot, no horse." Perhaps the number-one medical complaint horses have is hoof problems. Unlike the hooves of wild equids, those of domesticated horses are smaller, their walls more crumbly and prone to abscesses, white-line disease, and other problems that lead to lameness. Instead of using formaldehyde-based dressings, try adding supplements with biotin and methionine to the food or Chinese herbs that strengthen the Qi. My favorite is fo-ti (ho shu wu), because not only can it help hoof growth, it helps lower back pain and strengthens muscles, tendons, ligaments, and bones. If it is used with gotu kola, many of the effects of aging can be slowed. Fennel helps with absorption and digestion in general.

General Tonic Herbal Formula

The biggest problem with horses and herbs is that you need a lot of herbs to attain medicinal levels. This formula is cheap and effective. It can be obtained from a retailer of medicinal herbs for humans.

1 part fo-ti powder
1 part gotu kola powder
½ part fennel powder

Give a thousand-pound horse 1 ounce of mixture in his food daily, especially during cold winters. This formula works over time, so try it for at least a month. It is safe to give for the lifetime of the animal.

NATURAL MEDICINAL HERBAL GARDEN

These herbs are safe and easy to grow near the stables (where there is plenty of fertilizer!): comfrey, yarrow, broad-leaf plantain, calendula,

243

chamomile, and dandelion. Use these herbs in tea form by simmering ½ part herb to 2 parts water.

Comfrey: You can clean wounds with comfrey leaf and an antibiotic solution mixed together or even pack difficult-to-heal wounds with the fresh-ground leaves. I have seen the most amazingly stubborn wounds heal with minimal proud flesh. (Proud flesh is extra scar tissue that commonly proliferates on equine wounds.) Be sure not to confuse comfrey with highly toxic foxglove; the foliage looks similar.

Yarrow: An antimicrobial flower. Great to make into a tea and flush chronically infected wounds. Also, you can feed 1 cup of the flowers per day to aid in the treatment of strangles, which is a terribly contagious *Streptococcus* infection in the throat.

Plantain: Give as many of the leaves as your horse will eat to aid in the prevention of stress- or medication-induced gastric ulcers.

Calendula: Use the beautiful golden or orange flowers to aid in the treatment of wounds. Calendula, plantain, yarrow, and witch hazel make a wonderful tea for thrush.

Chamomile: To calm a horse down during travel, try a 60 cc syringe full of chamomile tea by mouth, or stir the warm tea into a small amount of bran mash. Chamomile flowers can be added dry into the grain or bran mash to aid in the soothing of the intestinal tract after long-term bute therapy.

Dandelion: After chronic medications or worming, help your horse's liver with as many dandelion leaves and flowers as he will eat.

Equine Herbal Distributors
- Hilton Herbs: 800-359-8076; www.hiltonherbs.com
- Dynamite Nutritional Supplements: www.dynamiteonline.com
- Advanced Biological Concepts—nutritional supplements: www.a-b-c-plus.com

For Early or Minor Colic
Colic is an illness specific to horses because they do not have the ability to vomit and their large, heavy colon has a tendency toward circulatory distress. In minor colic, the horse stops defecating, acts as if he is in pain, may paw or roll on the ground, and acts irritated. The intestinal motility signs are present but decreased. The heart rate and temperature are all normal (40 beats per minute, 99 degrees Fahrenheit). Veterinarians will often give

a Banamine injection and recommend walking the horse to try to increase peristalsis.

In severe colic, intravenous fluid and/or surgery may be required. The heart rate, temperature, and capillary refill time all are abnormal. You can tell that the capillary refill time is delayed when you press on your horse's gums and it takes a long time for the whitened fingerprint to become pink again. There are no gut sounds available. In an abdominal tap there may be high numbers of white blood cells, indicating leakage from the colon.

For any symptoms of colic, call your veterinarian. One of the best ways to prevent this disease is to make sure your horse has plenty of fresh, clean water and, ideally, consistently eats most meals of hay or grass. Bran mashes once a week help too. If your horse is prone to gas colic, try adding ½ cup of Colic Remedy to his bran mash (see page 233).

If colic does occur while the vet is in transit, walk your horse, choose a homeopathic from the list below, and give 3 to 5 pellets every fifteen minutes until the symptoms subside. Also do soft acupressure on the acupuncture point Stomach 2 slowly, massaging in a clockwise direction for ten minutes under both eyes. This point is about once inch under and to the midline of the medial canthus (or inner corner), right where the transverse facial vein divides.

TRY HOMEOPATHY

Nux vomica 30C: a general intestinal remedy useful especially if the horse has eaten too much; good to have in your first-aid kit

Arsenicum 30C: good if the horse has eaten rotten food and is pacing, restless but weak, wants company, or is thirsty

Rhus tox 30C: for a horse who is better walking and wants to walk

Bryonia 30C: for a horse who stays put, and will not move

China 30C: for a horse who shakes his head

Lycopodium 30C: for a horse with a very tense abdomen and who seems fearful of being left alone

Carbo vegetabilis 30C: for a horse with great abdominal distension, especially for impaction colic

Aconitum napellus 30C: for a horse who shows the first signs of pain, and is restless, rather angry, and violent, but hasn't sweated yet

245

Belladonna 30C: for a horse who is very hot, and sweaty, and whose heart you can feel beating when you touch any part of him

FARRIERY

Try Natural Balance shoeing techniques! They are based on Gene Ovnicek's study of wild horses' feet in their natural environment. This type of farriery brings the break-over point (from which the horse pushes off to begin his stride) farther back under the toe and helps provide load sharing through the back of the foot, as nature does, because the hoof is continually packed with dirt. This load sharing provides support to the internal structures of the foot while minimizing the forces exerted on the deep digital flexor tendon. Natural Balance farriery uses the coffin-bone position to determine the functional hoof angle. It is a science all its own. See www.hopeforsoundness.com or www.missionfarrieryschool.com.

THE BLACK LAB
WHO BRIDGED PHILOSOPHIES

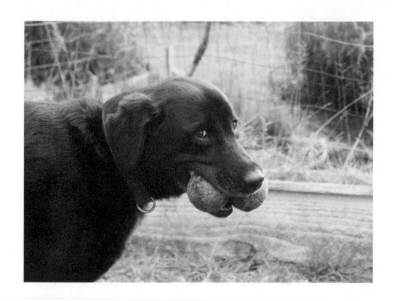

Zoe never dreamed that she would get into so much mischief, and I never expected that her case would help bring the worlds of Eastern and Western medicine together. During the long hours I treated her left hind leg, Zoe and I would look into each other's faces, eye to eye and nose to snout. The few black whiskers rose innocently, like eyebrows, each time I asked her, "Zoe, why are you so accident-prone?"

Perhaps the ten-year-old black Lab has always meant to be one of those quiet dogs everyone appreciates, who lies calmly in the corner. After all, her humans, Phil and Neave Megenhardt, have told me that she graduated from puppy obedience class as valedictorian. She impressed everyone by doing her "sits" and "stays" off-leash, while her puppy peers frantically scattered, following scents instead of obeying commands.

But Zoe has an uncanny knack for being in the wrong place at the wrong time. If there is broken glass to step on, a sharp bone to stick in the throat, or a fallen log to trip over, Zoe finds herself in the middle of it. When confronted with life's many temptations, all semblance of reason and safety escape her mind. The delights of stinky garbage, stray tennis balls, and pesky buzzing bees supersede the ever-fading memories of the inevitable sore tummy, sprained ankle, and swollen snout. That is why people love Zoe so much—she actually does what many of us wish we could do, hastily choosing temptation without a thought to the consequences.

Despite all her mishaps, an outsider might not notice any overt differences between Zoe and any other black Lab. But to those of us who know her, she has the distinguishing characteristics of an accident-prone canine. We recognize the signs of a dog living on the edge: teeth worn from too many rock-chewing sessions, missing nasal bones from being on the receiving end of a flying railroad spike, and surgical hardware in her rear leg from a mystery scrape with a concrete wall. Zoe has a medical record as thick as a telephone book.

The Megenhardts recognized early on that Zoe was going to be a problem dog. Being first-time dog parents, they could have avoided many of her earlier problems but learned how to prevent them too late. They decided to get pet insurance for Zoe. Even then, by some trick of nature, every time they let the coverage lapse, they were back at the vet's office for something else.

One of Zoe's most endearing hobbies was also one of her biggest problems. Zoe was an avid ball chaser. Once I threw a ball to her and she stood still, expectantly frozen, staring at me. I wondered what was wrong. Then Neave informed me that Zoe, overachiever that she is, will not chase a ball unless you throw two. She retrieves one and then somehow fits the second one in her mouth too. Even if both balls are floating in the water, Zoe will barge into the frigid lake to retrieve them, holding one in her mouth and searching for the second as if she is bobbing for apples. I will always think of Zoe with both green tennis balls stuffed skillfully into her mouth, proudly wagging her tail.

On Good Friday, when Zoe was only five months old—just a month after she ate feminine napkins and two months after she swallowed garden rocks again—the Megenhardts came home to find Zoe limping on her left hind leg. They wondered how she could have injured her leg after just a few hours in the yard by herself. Neave suspected some type of mishap with the concrete wall separating the yards. Phil suggested that the neighbors might have been involved. No one knew exactly how it had happened, but the veterinarian told them that she had managed to tear off a piece of the top of her left tibia bone right where the patellar ligament attaches. This is a very important piece of connective tissue that allows the knee to bend and straighten normally. Without the patellar ligament, Zoe would not be able to use her leg.

The veterinarian did surgery to stabilize Zoe's leg and she returned to normal. However, when she was almost five years old, the Megenhardts realized that something was wrong. It was a nice weekend day and Phil and Neave had just spent a year traveling, so to celebrate their return to Seattle, they took Zoe to an off-leash park. After throwing the dog both balls for a while, Neave suddenly heard horrific cries for help. She ran to see Zoe, rigid with pain, flopped on her back with her tail tucked tightly between her legs. The Megenhardts knew something truly awful had happened because, in addition to her high-pitched screaming, Zoe let both balls fall out of her mouth when she collapsed to the ground. Crippled with pain, the usually happy-go-lucky, sun-basking black Lab had to be carried to the car.

The Seattle family veterinarian did not feel comfortable treating Zoe's leg and referred the Megenhardts to a board-certified surgeon, Dr. Joe Battaglia, who has an excellent reputation. Neave had not known there were vets who spent four years in residency training programs and had to pass a rigorous exam in order to be certified in surgery. Still, in his thirty years of experience, Dr. Battaglia had never seen an injury like Zoe's.

Radiographs of Zoe's left knee revealed a bone-chilling finding—Dr. Battaglia saw a figure-eight-shaped piece of metal wire that should have been removed two weeks after the surgery, four years before. The original veterinarian made a grave mistake with young Zoe's leg. Not only did he leave the wire in, he also placed it too close to Zoe's growth plate, making normal bone development impossible.

The tibia had become deformed because it had grown around the wire, and it had also become very weak where the patellar tendon attached to it. The pull of the tendon finally snapped the top of the tibia off, the cause of Zoe's pain. Dr. Battaglia is a good surgeon, but even better, he applies an artist's inventive skill to the animals on his surgery table. The fate of Zoe's leg depended on his skillful approach and later upon my delicate acupuncture.

In April 1997, Dr. Battaglia removed the wire and rebuilt the top section of Zoe's tibia, a surgery he had never performed in his long career. Later, I looked at his thorough surgical records and drawings of each procedure. "Tibial crest transposition," the records say, complete with a detailed illustration that I examined for a long time. He included arrows showing vectors and biomechanical forces. *I wish I'd paid more attention in physics,* I thought. The pictures showed complicated turns and twists of metal, the sandwiching of a bone graft, and the screws holding it all in place.

Two months later, the records say, "Re-do tension band," and one month later, "Re-do allograft." After each written description Dr. Battaglia drew illustrations of each surgery. What the records didn't show was how frustrated and afraid he was that all her activity would rip his craftsmanship to pieces. Since Zoe is normally so active, it was difficult to keep her still between surgeries. It was necessary to keep the leg from moving so the bone would heal. After several months, this healing needed help, and that is when the Megenhardts found me.

I first saw Zoe and Neave in the fall of 1997. Zoe had spent several months in a cast, mostly in her small crate, and was still uncomfortable. In the exam room, she squirmed and whimpered when I touched the leg. I decided that in order to win her trust, the best thing to do was to first work on the muscle spasms in her back and on realigning her spine, because if I actually touched her swollen left knee, she winced. I showed Neave exercises to do on the left hind leg that would stretch the ligaments around Zoe's hock joint, now frozen from being in the cast for so long. Zoe tolerated that at least. Together we flexed the toes up and then folded them down to regain flexibility. I adjusted her spine and used my acupuncture-point-stimulating laser around her sore knee because she resisted needles. Then I prescribed a bone-and-ligament-healing herbal tea, a homemade diet, and numerous vitamin supplements.

The next time I saw Zoe, the Megenhardts had been told she was rejecting the bone graft. The small piece of bone Dr. Battaglia had screwed in place was slowly separating away. Although this piece was small, it was important because the patellar ligament attached to it. Every time the cast was removed, Neave rushed Zoe over for me to do acupuncture on the knee and then she rushed Zoe back to the surgeon for another cast application. After her six months of existing in a crate by day and in bed with Phil and Neave by night, Zoe's muscles had wasted away. The bones jutted out of her leg, hip, and pelvis, covered only by her shaved skin.

The Megenhardts held their beloved dog at night while she whimpered herself to sleep. They confided to me later that they desperately missed the bold fun-loving dog they had always known. Feeling guilty about having traveled for so long and being away from Zoe, Neave thought about her, years earlier, swimming in front of their kayaks, and how easily she had climbed aboard when she was tired. She thought about Zoe chasing stunt kites, racing beneath them and barking as they zoomed through the sky.

To Zoe, staying in a crate all day felt like jail, but it was a necessary evil. She was not allowed to run, jump, or even walk. Her whole personality shrank. Her spine shortened and humped. She contracted, tighter and tighter, until all the stress formed one large wrinkle in the middle of her forehead. Neave knew that "headache wrinkle" well because she began developing one too. It was as if the whole family bore the weight of trying to save Zoe's leg.

"I am afraid the leg must be amputated," the surgeon told them a few months after the second surgery seemed to have failed. Phil told me later that he was in shock. Everyone they talked to said the same thing—that Zoe would be fine without her leg. They said that her pain would cease and she would still be able to run.

Later, the Megenhardts told me what each of them thought. All Phil could hear was the disappearing thunder of Zoe's paws joyfully hitting the ground while they played ball. He wondered what three legs would sound like. While Phil felt determined to save Zoe's leg, Neave was thinking just the opposite. She wondered whether it was selfish to put Zoe through all this discomfort.

Strangely, the couple saw three-legged dogs everywhere they went that week. Small terriers, golden retrievers, poodles—you name the dog and the Megenhardts saw a three-legged version. By the end of the week, they had decided they'd try anything to save Zoe from amputation.

Faithfully, Neave came every few weeks for another appointment. I thought we might be able to save Zoe's leg, but little did I know how many obstacles there would be along the way. Over time, Zoe developed a spot where the cast rubbed that she licked incessantly. This is very common when casts have been on for a long time and the dog licks one pressure point. To me, it meant the nerves and blood supply were returning and may have felt tingly, like pins and needles. Acupuncture is very good for these "lick granulomas," and I decided to place the needles around the red, irritated sore, an ancient procedure called "surrounding the dragon."

Zoe was still far from being her ball-chasing former self, but Neave found a game they could play: the push-ball game. Neave would push a tennis ball at Zoe, and the dog would push it back. Although it was far from ball chasing, at least Zoe looked forward to it. She was feeling less pain and no longer needed to be held every night. She stopped whining and began walking around the house. After several acupuncture appointments, she was still very protective of her left leg. Sometimes she let me use moxibustion, the ancient technique of applying heated Chinese mugwort to the needles. Other times she wouldn't let me insert needles in the bad leg. During those sensitive times, I used my handheld laser to stimulate the points around her knee or lower down her leg at "ting" points, which restore Qi flow through each meridian.

Occasionally, Zoe would limp on another leg too. One day, she hobbled in limping on the right front leg, and of course also the left rear. "She jumped over a log before I could stop her," Neave said. Another time, Zoe had another strange accident with an exposed tree root or a fall down a hill, and had the swollen joint to prove it. I would change my points and treatment accordingly. One time she jammed a toe and needed a toe adjustment.

Slowly, week by week, her leg improved. It took many months to restore muscle tone and normal ability. Physical therapy and regular swimming helped strengthen and loosen her tendons and ligaments after so many months of being bound in a cast. Herbs helped alleviate the inflammation and pain by nourishing tissues. Chiropractic provided relief for Zoe too: As soon as she went home after an appointment, her contracted, hunched spine seemed to lengthen several inches. She slept all stretched out the way she used to.

I knew that without Dr. Battaglia's surgery skills, Eastern medicine alone would not have been enough to help Zoe. But I also knew that without holistic medicine, the surgery would have failed and Zoe would surely have lost her leg. Since holistic practitioners and surgeons treat one another's failures, how healthy animals would be if we could just forget mutual biases, combine medical philosophies, and respect one another.

Five years after Zoe's full recovery, Dr. Battaglia and I went out to lunch at the Jitterbug Café in Wallingford. We discussed Zoe and our sometimes differing views of medicine. Dr. Battaglia wore a purple Ocean Conservancy shirt and had his hair in a gray ponytail, and he spoke with a New Jersey accent. He had graduated from vet school in 1969, just two years after I was born!

Sipping an iced tea, he explained Zoe's surgery. "I placed the broken fragment farther up on the bone, where it is flatter and might accept the broken piece. I screwed it in place." He smiled with a childlike pride, describing his work as an architect or a sculptor would. "Then I did a bone-graft implantation around the fragment so it would adhere to the rest of the tibia," he said.

"But why did she need so many surgeries?" I asked over my beet salad, not to second-guess his work, but rather to better understand it.

"During the second surgery, I added more graft material. On the third and fourth surgeries, I loosened or tightened the screws, depending on how the radiograph looked, and changed her cast."

I looked at Dr. Battaglia's kind face. I knew so little about the way a surgeon must think, and I was pretty sure he knew nothing about the Gallbladder meridian, which transects both the hip and knee joints. But I also knew there was common ground: We both had helped Zoe. Instead of an acupuncture needle, he used a scalpel blade. Instead of understanding disease in terms of Qi-flow imbalances, he focused on a single area of pathology. Both philosophies were necessary.

As we spoke of Zoe's surgery, I had a vision of my grandmother strutting across the café floor with a cane in each hand. She stopped in front of our table, a mischievous gleam in her eye. Having been raised on a farm, she always told me, "You can judge just about anyone by his hands. Now look at Dr. Battaglia's large hands, thickened with calluses. Yep, we would have trusted him on the farm, because he has workin' hands—same as you." Both the surgeon and I use our hands to heal.

I remembered a story my friend Annie told me about Dr. Battaglia's hands. Her cat was bleeding internally and needed a splenic tumor removed. With blood transfusions, Dr. Battaglia performed the surgery, but he warned her ahead of time that his own hands were painful and faltering. "'I need surgery myself, and I just hope it is successful,'" Annie told me he said, lowering his eyes as he spoke, "'or I might not be able to do surgery anymore.'" She always remembered Dr. Battaglia's kindness and sincerity. A surgeon without functional hands is like an acupuncturist who's forgotten her Chinese meridians. Luckily, Dr. Battaglia's hand surgery was a success.

As open-minded as I was about his work, Dr. Battaglia gave me the impression that the feeling was not necessarily mutual. So I steered our conversation to the central point: Zoe Megenhardt would have needed an amputation without acupuncture. I knew it. The Megenhardts knew it. But would Dr. Battaglia admit it?

"Would you have predicted that Zoe could still walk so many years after surgery?" I asked. I wanted to tell him how excited I was to have reconnected Zoe's Gallbladder and Stomach meridians, which he had unknowingly transected during surgery. I wanted to show him my acupuncture needles, my electro-acupuncture machine, and the rest of my tools for healing. I wanted to invite him to work with me and talk to my clients, to hear their stories of how their pets were also healed with holistic medicine. Instead I silently waited for his response.

"No, she should have ruptured the patellar ligament a long time ago. I just don't understand it—the lag screw looks like it is hanging in midair." But it wasn't in midair, as we both knew, it was firmly embedded in scar tissue, which is not very visible on the films. To Dr. Battaglia, Zoe was some sort of anomaly, a freak of nature. He would have felt more comfortable if the screw were embedded in bone, as he had originally intended. I thought the explanation was that holistic medicine had provided the blood supply and helped the body build a powerful connective-tissue scar. Chinese needles helped with the pain. Comfrey herbal poultices on the hot, swollen knee joint healed the underlying tissues. This is the way healing has occurred for thousands of years, and now there was a remarkable surgeon in front of me dumbfounded by it.

"You know, that scar tissue is really solid. Dr. Bagley saw her and could not believe that she walks normally. No limp at all," I said. Dr. Rod Bagley is a well-respected neurosurgeon who went through veterinary acupuncture training and did an internship with me.

Dr. Battaglia and I left the café together and returned to our separate worlds. Over lunch I had felt that bridges were being formed, or the beginnings of them anyway. In the future, I would love to see Western and Eastern medical thoughts merge into single institutions and clinics. But I know there are obstacles.

Fear is a dangerous thing. It creates most of the misunderstandings in the world. Western doctors worry about what their peers would think and say if they embraced holistic medicine. Many of them believe only in double-blind studies, trials where neither the tester nor the testee know if they are receiving "real" treatment or a placebo. This type of experiment is impossible to perform with most types of holistic medicine because, of course, both tester and patient must be aware of a healing treatment. But as Dr. Battaglia pointed out, "Even open-heart surgery has never been proved in double-blind, placebo-controlled studies." Such studies would risk lives and be difficult to conduct, but obviously heart surgery is still a valid procedure. The same argument holds true for acupuncture.

A board-certified surgeon and a highly trained holistic veterinarian have one thing in common—they both build upon veterinary training. While there is an official exam surgeons need to pass to be board certified, no such thing exists yet for holistic veterinarians. It is unfortunate, but the public must do research to find out about a holistic veterinarian's training. Right now, anyone can say he or she is holistic; alone, it means very little.

Zoe is now eleven. It is as if she never had any surgeries; she is the most active dog of that age in my practice. That is, except when she is receiving acupuncture and chiropractic treatments, when she stands without moving for the entire half-hour session. Even with electric currents running between needles in her back and legs, she stands like a statue. Although she would rather be getting into mischief somewhere, she knows the treatments help her, and she cooperates so well that I can even busy myself with other tasks around the clinic and come back to find her motionless, acupuncture needles still in place.

Zoe still runs with two balls in her mouth, only occasionally resisting temptation. If she injures herself, she has a team of medical specialists that can help. If her back goes out and hunches, I am here to adjust her. If she loosens the screw holding her hind leg together, Zoe may need Dr. Battaglia to tighten it. And if she decides to eat a bee—again—Neave has a medical cabinet labeled "Zoe," with both Eastern and Western remedies inside.

❧

Zoe's Medicine Chest

Before your pet goes in for surgery, give him or her the homeopathic remedy *Arnica* 30C (see page 259). It is safe and effective to give the night before surgery, the morning of surgery, and for three days afterward. But have your vet check the stitches early. A lot of times stitches will become embedded when the animal is taking *Arnica,* because the tissue heals a lot faster than normal. If you need professional help with choosing remedies, contact www.ahvma.org for a list of holistic veterinarians. On this website, you can obtain information about a veterinarian's certification and interests.

Homemade diets best help pets recuperate from major surgery and debilitating illness. How are they supposed to improve without healthy building blocks?

Recuperation Gruel

1 cup low-sodium chicken broth
½ cup cooked oatmeal
¼ cup cooked chicken
1 mashed-up hard-boiled egg

Use a blender to make a liquidy gruel or slurry. Give a small amount at a time as directed by your veterinarian.

Comfrey Packs

After the stitches are out, to help with inflammation and swelling, grind up some fresh comfrey leaves and pour hot water over them. Then drain off the water, leaving the softened leaves. Take the warm herbal mush into your hands and hold it against the affected area for 10 minutes twice a day.

Hot-Spot Relief Tea

Many pets lick at the surgery site or lick due to skin allergies. An easy thing to do with hot spots, no matter what the cause, is to hold a moistened or used black tea bag on the site for 10 minutes twice a day. This more complicated herbal formula will work on difficult hot spots. Do not use supercold compresses on the spot, because it is extremely sensitive and can be quite painful.

2 quarts fresh-bottled or filtered water
½ cup calendula flowers (fresh is best—easy to grow!)
¼ cup chamomile flowers (ditto)
¼ cup yarrow flowers (ditto)
¼ cup comfrey leaves
¼ cup grindelia flowers
⅛ cup plantain leaves
2 tablespoons goldenseal powder (an antimicrobial herb)

Combine all of the ingredients in a stainless steel or ceramic saucepan, cover, and simmer over low heat for 10 minutes. Remove from the heat, uncover, and let cool and steep for about 2 to 3 hours. Strain the tea, discarding the solids. Warm the tea to room temperature for each application. Apply tea with a cotton ball to the hot spot for 10 minutes 2 to 4 times a day for 3 days. If it does not improve within 1 day, go back to your veterinarian.

Keeping: The tea will last for up to 3 weeks in the refrigerator. You can also freeze it in an ice cube tray, and thaw as needed.

INSECT-STING THERAPY

If a dog gets stung by a bee or spider, sometimes the only way to tell is by his swollen face. If you see this, you should give 25 milligrams of Benadryl by mouth. It is also a good idea to go to the veterinarian. Sometimes that swelling can cause trouble with breathing, which is much more serious. The homeopathics *Ledum* 30C and *Apis* 30C alternated every 10 minutes might also be beneficial on the way to the veterinarian.

HEALING FOR TRAUMA

This section applies to all animals.

Arnica 30C. This is the best-known remedy for any type of trauma. The dog may have a sore spot that is very sensitive to the touch. The animal may want to lie down but shifts sides or moves from one spot to another frequently. Give 3 pellets once, either dry in the mouth or mixed with water and spooned into the mouth.

Hypericum 30C. This remedy will be helpful for trauma to the toes, such as when a dog is stepped on; your dog may be limping and a veterinarian has determined that there is no fracture. Give 3 pellets twice a day for 3 days.

Symphytum 30C. Give to speed up bone healing, 3 pellets twice a day for 5 days.

EAR PROBLEMS

Yeast and bacteria are a problem in dogs and cats that have a tendency to store Damp Heat along the Triple Heater meridian. Diet changes and vitamins can help. A good all-around ear cleanser is a mixture of 1 part white vinegar to 9 parts water. Dip a cotton ball in the solution and clean the ears with it weekly. For infections, my favorite medication is enzymatic—containing no antibiotics—and is called Zymox (see page 264).

FEAR AND ANXIETY DURING STORMS

Phosphorus 30C. The dog shakes and trembles and looks at you as if asking for help. This is usually a very affectionate dog who loves and is loved by everybody. Give 3 pellets at the first sign of a storm.

Silica 30C. The animal gets very exited before the storm, as if she were happy. During the storm, she shakes and seeks company. This is a dog of mild temperament that "never does anything wrong" and is very set in her routines. Give 3 pellets at the first sign of an approaching storm.

Aconitum 30C. The dog is extremely agitated and may bark and move about. His or her eyes may seem bigger than normal. Give 3 pellets at the first sign of an approaching storm.

Relaxation Medley

Good for dogs, cats, and birds during firework season, thunderstorms, traveling, or other times of stress. Also see below for homeopathic remedies for behavioral problems.

2 quarts low-sodium chicken broth or water
⅓ cup passionflower
⅓ cup chamomile flowers
¼ cup cut oatstraw leaves and stems
¼ cup packed hops flowers
¼ cup scullcap leaves
⅓ cup lobelia leaves
1 tablespoon powdered kava kava

Combine all of the ingredients in a stainless steel or ceramic saucepan, cover, and simmer over low heat for 20 minutes. Remove from the heat, uncover, and allow to set for at least 6 hours. The dose is 1 tablespoon per 25 pounds of body weight. An average cat weighs

10 pounds and would get ½ tablespoon. A bird would get 1 milliliter per kilogram on a piece of cracker, so the average cockatoo gets about 0.4 milliliter. Give the tea 2 to 3 times a day, depending on how stressed your pet is. It takes about 2 hours to take effect and should not cause overt sedation. It should relieve the fright and agitation.

SADNESS/GRIEF

Ignatia amara 30C. This remedy may help a dog that is showing signs of sadness, including social withdrawal. The symptoms usually start after the loss of a playmate or because his or her favorite human has gone away. Give 3 pellets 3 times at 12-hour intervals.

RESOURCES

For Chinese extract granulated herbs:
  KPC Herbs, 800-KPC-8188; www.kpc.com
  Golden Flower, 800-729-8509; www.gfcherbs.com
  Brion, 800-333-4372

For Chinese patents, Chinese raw herbs for teas:
  Mayway, 800-2-MAYWAY; www.mayway.com

For *Lithospermum* 15 and other formulas based on patent Chinese herbals:
  ITM, 800-544-7504; www.itmonline.org

For Western herbs for powders or raw herbs for teas (remember, your herbs should be fresh—alfalfa powder bright green, goldenseal root powder rich yellow):
  Western Herbs, P.O. Box 115, 21627 Sertz Road, Index, WA 98256;
    800-274-4372
  Frontier Herbs, 800-669-3275; www.frontierherb.com
  Wise Woman Herbals, 235 N. Mill, Unit A, Cresswell, OR 97426;
    541-895-5152
  Trinity Herbs, P.O. Box 1001, Graton, CA 95499; 888-874-4372;
    www.trinityherbs.com (wholesale only)
  Jean's Greens, 119 Sulphur Spring Road, Norway, NY 13416;
    315-845-6500; www.jeansgreens.com
  Healing Spirits, 9198 State Route 415, Avoca, NY 14809; 607-566-2701;
    www.infoblvd.net/healingspirits
  Animals' Apawthecary Co., P.O. Box 1645, Hamilton, MT 59840;
    406-375-8145; apawlab@montana.com
  Mountain Rose Herbals, 85472 Dilley Lane, Eugene, OR 97405;
    800-879-3337; www.mountainroseherbs.com

For Ayurvedic herbs:
  Banyan, 800-953-6424; www.banyanbotanicals.com
    They have a great "Heart Formula" I use for early cardiac disease or
    when there is a severe heart murmur; helps prevent congestive heart
    failure.
  Ayush, 425-637-1400; www.ayush.com

For homeopathic medicines (specify tiny granules for animals):
  Dolisos, 800-877-8038; www.dolisos.com
  Washington Homeopathics, 800-336-1695
  Boiron, 800-BOIRON-1; www.boiron.com

For Prozyme, a fantastic enzyme source for chronic digestive problems:
  1-800-522-5537

For flower essences (emotional support for pets and their owners):
  Green Hope Farm, 603-469-3662; www.greenhopeessences.com
  Energetic Essences Elixirs, 505-586-1607; www.petessences.com

For amazing enzymatic ear medication called Zymox (for dogs and cats):
  Pet King, 630-241-3905; www.petkingbrands.com/zymox.html

  Contact the Veterinary Botanical Medical Association (www.vbma.org)
  for information on the use of herbal medicines in the treatment of animals.

RECOMMENDED BOOKS

For Medical Information

Fox, Michael W. *The Healing Touch: The Proven Massage Program for Cats and Dogs.*
Reissue ed. New York: Newmarket Press, 1990.
  Dr. Michael Fox has written many books. I spoke to him when I was considering working with his animal welfare project in India. We are fortunate
  to have such a kind activist, and so are the animals!

Goldstein, Martin. *The Nature of Animal Healing: The Path to Your Pet's Health,
Happiness, and Longevity.* New York: Alfred A. Knopf, 1999.
  I love Dr. Marty's diet information and his overall positive attitude.

Poutinen, C. J., and Beverly Cappel-King. *The Encyclopedia of Natural Pet Care.*
2nd ed. New York: McGraw-Hill, 2000.

Schwartz, Cheryl. *Four Paws, Five Directions: A Guide to Chinese Medicine for Cats and Dogs*. Berkeley, Calif.: Celestial Arts, 1996.
Dr. Cheryl is simply amazing as a holistic veterinarian, teacher, mentor, and windsurfer.

Segal, Monica. *K9 Kitchen, Your Dog's Diet: The Truth Behind the Hype*. Toronto: Doggie Diner, 2002.

Snow, Amy, Nancy Zidonis, Ella Bittel, and Carla Stroh. *The Well-Connected Dog: A Guide to Canine Acupressure*. Denver: Tallgrass Publishers, 1999.
Ella Bittel and I go way back. We taught the IVAS acupuncture course together and we trained with the AVCA together. She has worked on my own horse. This book and its equine version have received great reviews.

Wulff-Tilford, Mary L., and Gregory L. Tilford. *All You Ever Wanted to Know About Herbs for Pets*. Irvine, Calif.: Bowtie Press, 1999.
I met Greg and Mary at an American Herbalist Guild conference and they are as sweet as they are knowledgeable.

Wynn, S., and S. Marsden. *Manual of Natural Veterinary Medicine: Science and Tradition*. St. Louis: Mosby, 2002.

For the Human/Animal Bond

McElroy, Susan Chernak. *Animals as Guides for the Soul*. Reissue ed. New York: Ballantine Books, 1999.

McElroy, Susan Chernak. *Animals as Teachers and Healers*. Reissue ed. New York: Ballantine Books, 1998.

Schoen, Allen. *Kindred Spirits*. New York: Broadway Books, 2001.
Allen was kind enough to take me as an intern even though I knew next to nothing about acupuncture. He is a magical force when it comes to helping animals. Once, at night, we were driving down a busy four-lane street in Seattle and two dogs jumped in front of the car. Of course, one had to be a golden retriever (Allen's favorite breed), so he demanded that I pull over immediately and he jumped into traffic to save them. I sat on the sidelines praying and calling the dogs. All I could hear was people asking, "Who was that woman who didn't stop him from getting hurt?" Luckily everyone got out of the road safely.

HOW TO FIND A HOLISTIC PRACTITIONER IN YOUR AREA

For general information and referrals: www.ahvma.org
It is not necessary to have attained any certification or extra education to belong to this association, but through this website you can research the credentials of holistic-minded veterinarians.

For veterinarians specializing in acupuncture: IVAS, P.O. Box 1478, Longmont, CO 80502; 303-682-1167; www.ivas.org; office@ivas.org

For veterinarians specializing in chiropractic: AVCA, 623 Main Street, Hillsdale, IL 61257; 309-658-2920; www.avcadoctors.com

For veterinarians specializing in homeopathy: www.theavh.org

For veterinarians specializing in herbal treatments: www.vbma.org
There are many programs available in Chinese and Western herbal medicine. It is best to ask your veterinarian about his or her training.

For veterinarians specializing in NAET allergy and pain treatment: www.naet.com

For veterinarians specializing in T-touch massage technique: www.tteam-ttouch.com

For veterinarians specializing in Bowen therapy: www.bowtech.com

ACKNOWLEDGMENTS

I thank my mother, Ann Kelleher, who is a political science professor and taught countless college students, as she taught me, that, depending upon one's cultural origin, there are many facets of reality. When I grew up, visitors from all over the world stayed with us—among them a Thai man who rescued child prostitutes and provided career training, a British service worker, and a Norwegian woman whose mission was to form a partnership with a college in Namibia. These visitors thought differently from me, they ate differently (once we spent the day searching for soy milk before it was popular in America), and they came from countries my mother had visited but that I could only wonder about. Through my mother's international work and, especially, from her insight, I was taught that often I had much to learn from the world's people, at times even more than from my own university professors. That learning would open my mind to the medical philosophies of other nations.

I wish to thank Mary Ann Naples, my beloved agent, whose commitment and compassion for animals could not run deeper. Thanks also to editing whiz Amanda Katz for her fine work. How can anyone write so small? And to Beth Wareham, my editor at Scribner, and Rica Allannic.

To all my patients and to their people. The psychic connection between pets and their people will never cease to amaze me—like Jan Johnson and her cat, Romeo; and Eric Paulsen with his fluffy kitty, Katie.

I want to thank Dr. Mike Flaherty, who introduced me to Brenda Peterson. Without Brenda, there would be no book. Through her writing classes and the input of my fellow writers and animal activists such as Ward Serrill, Leigh Calvez, Vanessa Adams, and Jackie Bergmann (who took the photograph of Tiger Lily on page 143), I continue to develop my writing craft. Thank you to my partner, photographer, and website builder, Nabeel Daniel Seirawan.

Thanks to Dr. Tracy Bennett, whose empathy for and vast knowledge of birds and exotic pets is an inspiration to all who know her. Dr. Adawna Windom, who helped me lift Kade, the 120-pound epileptic dog, onto her surgery table for gold bead implants. The naturopathic veterinary whiz Dr. Steve Marsden, who has helped hundreds of cancer patients holistically. Thank you to Dr. Mike Lemmon, who was one of the first holistic vets in the States. As an American soldier in Korea, he opened up to natural medicines after meeting monks in the mountains who cleansed his burdened mind. Thanks to Dr. Susan Wynn, who keeps us on the conventional scientific path. And to all the vets who practice medicine with their hearts as well as their minds. Fixing animals is not always easy; they can't talk, so we have to learn to *read* them.

To my other teachers: Mrs. Henderson and Ms. Watson from Bartlett Elementary School in Malden, Massachusetts (circa 1978); without my one year at Bartlett, I wouldn't be able to write at all. Dr. David Mizamoto from Drew University for spurring my interest in slime molds. Dr. Veronica Kiklivich and Drs. Steve and Melissa Hines from the College of Veterinary Medicine at Washington State University for infusing a touch of practicality into the curriculum. Herbal teachers Michael Pilarski for teaching sustainable wild harvesting, Adrienne Roan Bear for her unique spiritual connection with healing plants, and Karta Purkh Singh Khalsa for awesome herbal knowledge. Iridologist Jivan Swann for teaching me how to read the body through the eyes. Teaching is the grandest gift for our future.

For awesome peer review and editing: Dr. Jean Dodds, Dr. Christine Susumi, Dr. Tracy Bennett for the information on general avian care, Dr. Naomi Bierman, Dr. Rob Echentile, Dr. Jackie Obando, Dr. Fernando Moncayo, Dr. Tamara Norquist, and Dr. Tina Ellenbogen. Thanks to Dr. Erin Zamzow, Dr. Jane Koepcke, and surgeon Dr. Karl White at WSU for pushing for an alternative surgery program. I want to thank my dad, Bill Kelleher, my brother, Neil Kelleher, and the rest of my wonderful family. And Diane, Irene, and Linda at Sudden Printing in West Seattle for just being nice.

I long for the day the power of the pharmaceutical industry shrinks to reasonable proportions because people learn to take control of their own healing. I wish to thank my heroes Michael Moore and Michael Moore—the herbalist and the working person's activist. I also wish for a time when books are printed on hemp paper to save trees.

INDEX

ABOUT THE AUTHOR

Donna Kelleher, D.V.M., graduated from Washington State University College of Veterinary Medicine. While still training as a senior veterinary student, she entered an internship with her mentor, Allen Schoen, author of *Love, Miracles, and Animal Healing,* which led to her securing a scholarship in veterinary acupuncture. Today, Dr. Kelleher is certified by the International Veterinary Acupuncture Society and American Veterinary Chiropractic Association and uses chiropractic in combination with acupuncture, herbs, and nutrition to heal animals. She is president of the Washington chapter of the American Holistic Veterinary Medical Association, and through her efforts this chapter was one of the first in the country to be accepted as a chapter of a local conventional veterinary association. She is a vegan and loves gardening.